BONE MEDICINE

BONE MEDICINE

Native American Guide to Physical Wholeness

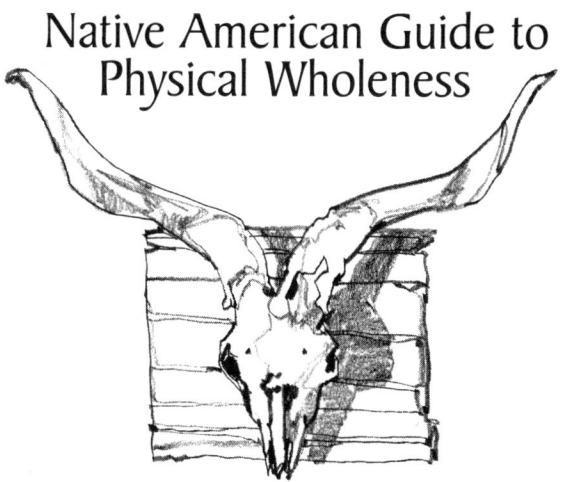

Wolf Moondance

Illustrated by Jim Sharpe and Sky Starhawk

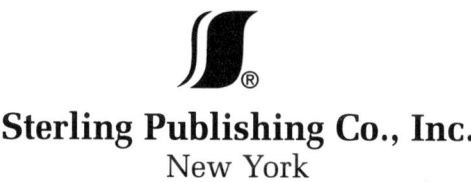

Sterling Publishing Co., Inc.
New York

Library of Congress Cataloging-in-Publication Data
Moondance, Wolf.
Bone medicine : a Native American shaman's guide to physical wholeness / Wolf Moondance ; illustrated by Jim Sharpe & Sky Starhawk.
    p. cm.
ISBN 0-8069-9797-4
1.Medicine wheels—Miscellanea. 2. Spiritual life. I. Title.
BF1623.M43M65 1999
299'.7-dc21   99-12226
                                                                CIP

    10 9 8 7 6 5 4 3 2 1

Published by Sterling Publishing Company, Inc.
387 Park Avenue South, New York, N.Y. 10016
© 1999 by Wolf Moondance
Additional illustrations © 1999 by Jim Sharpe
Distributed in Canada by Sterling Publishing
c/o Canadian Manda Group, One Atlantic Avenue, Suite 105
Toronto, Ontario, Canada M6K 3E7
Distributed in Great Britain and Europe by Cassell PLC
Wellington House, 125 Strand, London WC2R 0BB, England
Distributed in Australia by Capricorn Link (Australia) Pty Ltd.
P.O. Box 6651, Baulkham Hills, Business Centre, NSW 2153, Australia
Manufactured in the United States of America
All rights reserved

Sterling ISBN 0-8069-9797-4

*To Liz—
everyone should be so blessed as to have a Mom Liz.
You and Dad Jim are Home,
and there is no place like home...
To you, Liz!!!*

Other books by the same author:

RAINBOW MEDICINE

SPIRIT MEDICINE

STAR MEDICINE

Contents

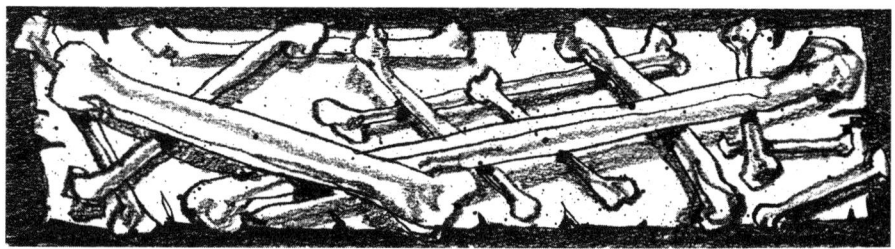

Acknowledgments   9

Purpose   11

1. Sacred Circles   16
   Personal Journal
   Physical Medicine Teachings
   Medicine Blanket
   Making Prayer Ties
   Ceremony of Sacred Herbs
   How to Build a Rainbow Medicine Wheel

2. The Gateway of the West (Circle of the Bear)   35
   Ceremony of Introspection
   Ceremony of Intention
   Spiritual Colors of the Physical Movements
   Teachings of Acceptance

3. Old Woman Rock—Nurture   51
   Teachings of Nurture—Cougar Medicine
   Life Circles—Ceremony of Connecting the Spirit and the Physical
   Physical Medicine Bundle
   Process of the Lesson of Purpose—Teachings of the Dragon

4. The Turn in the Road—Choice   67
   Teachings of Choice—Raven Medicine
   Ceremony of Choice—The Broken Stick Ceremony of Forgiveness
   Ceremonial Medicine Pouch of the West
   Process of the Lesson of Obedience—Bat Medicine

5. The Wind's Voice—Ceremony   88
   Teachings of Ceremony—Ladybug Medicine
   Ceremonial Stick

Ceremony of Light
Process of the Lesson of Life—Teachings of the Human Being

6. Snake Man's Vision—Change   **105**
Teachings of Change—White-Tailed Deer Medicine
Ceremony of the Cleansing of the Physical Body
Process of the Lesson of Action—Teachings of the Mule Deer

7. Talking Bones—Proof   **124**
Teachings of Proof—Fox Medicine
Ceremony of the Breath of Life
Ceremonial Water Bowl
Process of the Lesson of Solid—Crow Teachings

8. The Song of the Bones—Real   **139**
Teachings of Real—Skunk Medicine
Ceremony of the Tree of Real
Process of the Lesson of Full—Ant Teachings

9. The Golden Door—Grand   **152**
The Teachings of Grand—Ram Medicine
Ceremony of Grandness
Shaman's Necklace
Process of the Lesson of Worthy—Lynx Teachings
Ceremony of Worthy

10. The Call of the Wolf   **168**
Ceremony of the Five Colored Horses
Ceremony of the White Wolf

Rainbow Totem and Guide Teachings   **181**
Medicine Word Interpretations
Lesson Word Interpretations
Herbs
Animal Guides and Totems
Mineral Medicines
Colors

Index   **189**

ACKNOWLEDGMENTS

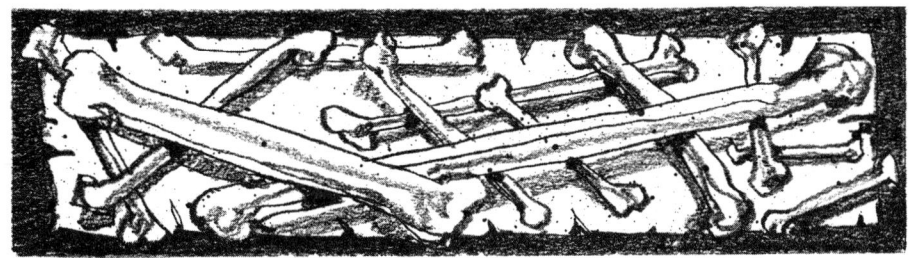

There have been those in my life who have opened doors for me, and I would like to acknowledge the inspiration, the intensity, the impeccability, and the spirituality that brought a physical change to my existence. You, each one of you that follow, are those:

All my students, everyone who has ever studied with Wolf Moondance, thank you. My heartfelt gratitude goes to Lil Westbrook, William R. Brown, Margaret J. Willis, Anita Bilby, and Gerald W. Harman. Your physical existence while you walked two-legged on this earth gave me direction. You were my grandma, you were my uncle, you were my sister, you were my poppy, you were my student. You taught me that life is giving to other people; life is getting from other people; life is a circle. As you have crossed from the physical plane, you now speak to me always as spirit. Thank you.

I have a very special hug for four very special people: Phyllis and Pete—you are grand, grand parents. Pete, you directed my life in such a way that I have found home.

My gratitude is even larger than usual for Sheila Anne Barry. This time I can't just say "Thank you, Sheila." It's time to get real in this book, and a rewrite sometimes isn't a bad thing. Thank you, thank you, thank you. In everything we do we need a mom, and like I've always said, you are my mom when it comes to writing. I listen and I try, and I do. God bless.

Joanne—thanks for your magic fingers, and the rewrite. But more than anything, you are one of the best daughters this shaman has ever had. You stand in a place where things are physical now, a place where you have been a student and are a teacher. It's time, Granny Jo.

My heartfelt gratitude and great admiration always goes to my mother. I know, Mom, that heaven is real. Thank you.

There are times in our lives when we need a doctor, and I have had some wonderful ones in my life. There are times in our lives when we need teachers, and I have had some wonderful ones.

Body workers are necessary in our physical existence and I only know one good one. From Mom Wolf, Lael, you are the answer to pain. You scatter stars of truth and teach those lessons in wonderful ways. We must breathe, we must sing, we must play, and we must feel. You carry that always as your sacred medicine, and I acknowledge you with great honor and respect. Congrats on a wonderful son.

Much love to my brother-in-law, Troy. You are the grandest dad that my nephew could have had, the best half-side to my sister, and I know the best friend that I've had, because you speak truth. Sometimes it is painful, but always it is truth. My love to my brother Jim; the lessons go on!

No acknowledgment is complete without a thank you to my half-side. Raven, this is the year 44. The lake, the sunset, four books. Thanks for the support.

Aho.

PURPOSE

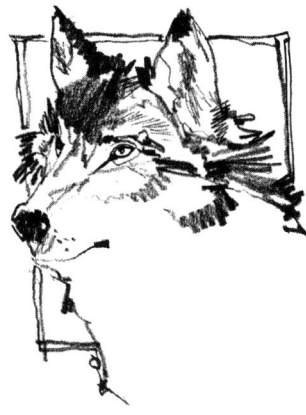

At a young age, I was given a vision of the sun and a crescent moon and seven stars—one each of red, orange, yellow, green, blue, purple, and burgundy. From that vision I connected with a very old teaching known as the Medicine Wheel. After I had seen several medicine wheels, I realized that the wheel was a place of learning. It was a place where you could go and hold hands with Great Spirit. You could learn, in other words. I placed my vision in the physical plane by connecting it with the stones of a medicine wheel. Those stones create a school I call the Sacred Mystery School. A mystery school is a place where mysteries are revealed.

The school that I take care of, and have been given the privilege of being a caretaker of, is known as the school of Rainbow Medicine, or the Rainbow Medicine Wheel.

The Rainbow Medicine Wheel has four sections, with a center and a cross. Each stone and each portion of that cross, and each part of the center, is a lesson or a medicine. We are now in the third level of the Rainbow Medicine Wheel—and this book is called "Bone Medicine" for the physical section of the medicine wheel. The first section is Spirit, the second section is Emotion, the third section is Physical, the fourth section is the Mind. The cross formed by the lines running between East and West, and North and South, divides the inner portion of the circle into sections. These are the lessons in life. They are known as the Red and Blue Roads. We walk that Red Road, we walk that Blue Road. The Red Road represents the lessons of spirit, and the Blue Road the lessons of physicality. The center of the Rainbow Medicine Wheel is called the "Song of Great Spirit." It consists of seven stones that make a circle, with an eighth stone in the center. The center stone represents Creator and the circle around it is the song of the Creator.

Bone Medicine is a book about life. In this book of life, you are given opportunities to learn the seven sacred medicines of physicality—which are Nurture, Choice, Ceremony, Change, Proof, Real, and Grand. You are given the opportunity to learn the seven lessons in this section, which are *purpose, obedience, life, action, solid, complete,* and *worthy.*

It is such an interesting life that you could write books about each one of those words. I will bring the Medicine Wheel to life within this book. I will show you physical ways to respect, to obey, to appreciate, and to accept your physical existence. There is shamanism in this book. There can't be anything in life that doesn't contain shamanism, for shamanism is a connection between the physical world and the spiritual world—and there is nothing in our existence that shamanism is not a part of. You can exchange the word "shaman" or "shamanism" with the word "spirituality." You can exchange the word "unique," "supernatural, "or "individual" with the word "shaman" or "shamanic." One of the more powerful words that you will experience while reading this book is the word "journey." Each chapter starts out with a spiritual shamanic journey. This allows you to connect the spirit world with the real world. Many times I have been asked by my readers, "Did this really happen?" Each time you have a shamanic journey, you have a shaman's understanding of physical existence and spiritual opportunity. Yes, these visions really happened, and yes, there are really things that happen in physicality that connect to the spiritual.

My strongest purpose in this book is to help you understand your physical wholeness. Physicality is opportunity. We are a sacred circle when we live a human wholeness. We are never separated from the spirit. We are not a broken hoop; we are not defeated. We are not destroyed; we are not a dead race. We are alive and we have opportunity. Within the Rainbow Medicine Wheel you connect with the spirit world through spirit guides. You make connections on each level of the Medicine Wheel with spirit guides, with teachers and ancestors from the spirit world who make their presence known in a very physical way in your life. They give you opportunity.

In this section of the Rainbow Medicine Wheel you will encounter the bat, dragon, human, antelope, crow, ant, lynx, cougar, raven, ladybug, deer, fox, skunk, and ram. They are animal totems, two-legged totems, crawly totems, winged totems—they are totems that connect you and guide you to your physical opportunity and bring you a better understanding from the realm of spirit.

I hope to share my Native Americanism with you through an understanding that we are all one circle. My question is, what color is a circle? Time's up—the answer to the question is, a circle has no color. It has form. First and foremost, a circle is a form—a shape, in other words. Now you can paint it black or you can paint it white, or you can paint it green, if you want to, and then there would be a race of green people. There is: they are people who don't know anything yet, and they are just getting started. They are on the road to growth. A green person is either someone who is eaten up with envy or someone who is brand new. But when we get down to the truth, has anyone ever seen a green person? Well, if we watch TV we have. So life can be very confusing. It can have its pitfalls and sadness, and those all involve emotions. That takes us to the second section of the wheel. It also allows us to be in the mental plane, for everything we do and everything we are, is a thought. When we study the Medicine Wheel, things are deep—not lightweight. They are an experience.

When I took English in school, I didn't learn anything because I couldn't understand the limitation of words. Words are not words to me—they are spirits. Every word we have has been classified as a noun, a pronoun, an adjective, and so on. That's not what words are to me. Words are feelings, feelings are thoughts, thoughts are emotions, emotions are energy, energy is spirit, and spirit is everything. If you didn't like that sentence, you probably won't like this book—or any other book I write—because my challenge as a shaman is to get you to live in two worlds at one time. Then you are a total circle, night and day, up and down, back and forth. If you like that, then your spirituality is shamanism.

Now that doesn't make shamanism your religion, because there is no worship involved in it. Shamanism is a way of life that is based on an understanding of communication with the spirit world. It is daily discipline that you receive from the spirit and apply to actions in your life. Shamanism is both worlds: the physical Blue Road and the spiritual Red Road.

You will encounter the lessons and medicines of the physical section of the Rainbow Medicine Wheel and you will experience a journey that I have been on since I was five years old. My mother passed on to me, her oldest daughter, shamanism. She gave me an understanding of my native heritage. I am a mixed blood, a biracial baby. I have rainbow blood, which gives me the opportunity to belong to all people. Many people base a lot on a bloodline. I base a lot on heart. What color we are—or what race we are—is not always truth, and I feel our physical should be truth—truth that we are all two-leggeds and of one race—"the human race."

My point in this book is to achieve physical wholeness—for us to say simply, "I am a human being," to understand that we are one circle (one people, too), and accept that we all are the sacred hoop of mankind. Physical wholeness is an opportunity, an adventure, a journey—it's life, and life is intense. Life is full of zest, full of spirit, and it houses itself within a physical form known as matter, muscle, blood, bone, DNA, tissue.

At first, in the writing of this book, I felt tremendous anguish trying to explain the two-legged experience. Then I realized that all I needed to do was to sit back and tell what I know in my heart, for that is Native. So many people today are looking for Native American teachings. Let me give you a really big one—it is heart, it is family, and that is a circle. It has gone on from mother to daughter, from father to son, from the sun and the moon, from light and dark, up and down. If you understand that, then you know what Native American is.

But we're not just Native American, we're Lakota, Apache, Iroquois—we have our bands. If I knew other bloods, I would know that they have their bands too. Scots have their clans; Celts have theirs. There are different types of Jewish families. There are different kinds of African blood. They aren't only African—they're Jamaican, African-American, Egyptian.

In the physical section of the Rainbow Medicine Wheel you have to get real, and the way you get real is to achieve the core. There will be pain when that happens, because there will be growth. Just remember there is no gain without pain and there is no pain without gain. When we open our eyes and listen to Old Woman Rock, and we take the turn in the road that is Choice, we give ourselves a wonderful opportunity to celebrate Ceremony. Ceremony brings about Change, and that

Change is the outcome, which is Proof. That is one of the most Grand things you can do in life. You are nurturing yourself at that point. Our physicality gives us a chance to know that we are spirit, because life is not limited by death. Our existence doesn't end when we die and it doesn't begin when we die. In a circle there is no beginning and no end. There never was a beginning and there never will be an end. That is hard for our small minds to grasp, but expand yourself: Think of everything you do in life as an adventure, an experience. Our life is a spiritual trip. We are spirits with the chance to smell, hear, feel, and be. We are human beings—the journey of physical existence.

Aho.

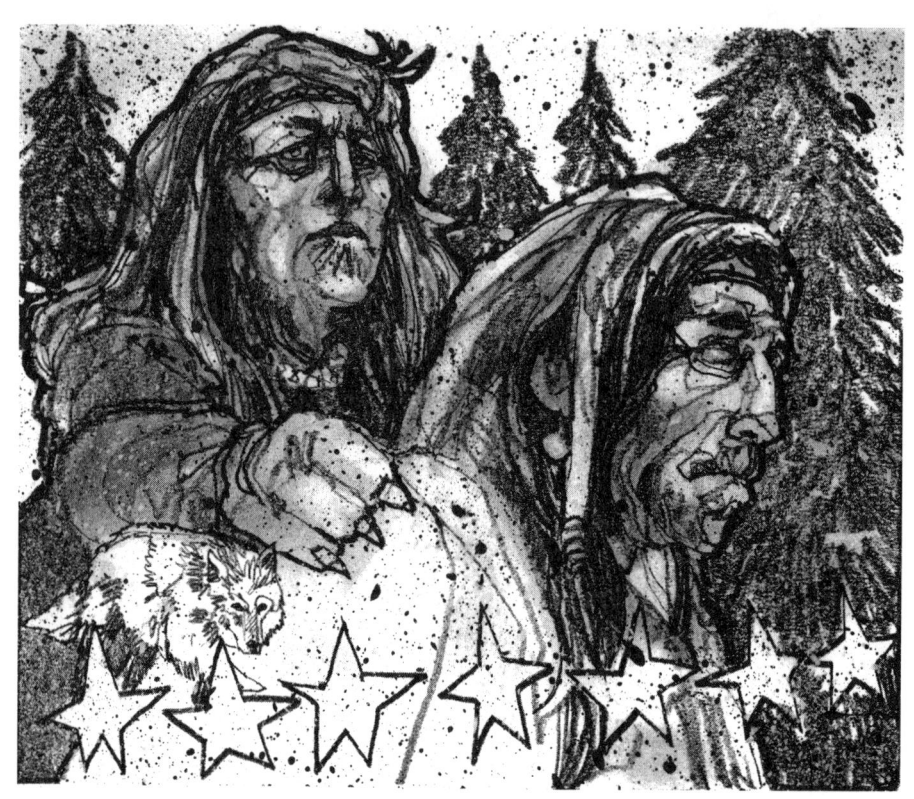

1
SACRED CIRCLES

Night has come a few minutes before seven. It is Fall and I can smell the earth. A soft misty rain falls gently. Fall is a wonderful time with the black silhouettes of trees pressing their bodies against the flaming orange sky. Seven eager students are approaching and I, once again, have been asked to be their Wolf. To guide them, to teach them—that will be my path. I stand at the East gate. In front of me is the Medicine Wheel—a wheel of rainbow colors, of rocks in all seven colors. I spiral in, raising my hand and giving thanks to Great Spirit, Grandmother/Grandfather.

"Here I am again, Grandmother/Grandfather, and it is time. I must teach the physical section of the wheel."

Standing in front of the West gate I see the blue flag blowing in the wind. Seven medicine stones and seven words—seven lesson words, seven stones. I take a deep breath and look through the West gate. Soft wet grass lies before me. Familiar smells of Fall—rain and earth I smell. All around me it's becoming noisy: I hear twinkling sounds, clattering and clicking, rattling, clanging, jingling sounds. There is a symphony of noise that spins around me, and I see colors watching over me. Tiny points of light. My thoughts fill my mind.

I sit and lean back against a tall ponderosa pine. I breathe in and out, and relax. I have the obligation to teach. That obligation is a job and that job is shaman. There is no fear, for my mother has instilled a knowing that resonates deep from within my spirit. I take a deep breath, lift my chin to the sky, and exhale. But I'm just a human. I'm lower than the dirt itself for I have sin and I hurt people and I fall short every day of being perfect.

"Yes, Granddaughter, you do," a familiar voice says. "But are you going to take them on this special journey and teach them sacred circles?"

"Yes, it's your opportunity," a stronger voice says, and they both appear in front of me—Grandmother and Grandfather Wolf.

I can feel that special twinkling, tingling. I can smell home—the fragrance of the river, the beauty of the flowers, the sounds of soft water trickling over the rocks. The gentle breeze caresses the cottonwood trees.

"Now, Granddaughter," Grandmother says. "Do you want to teach the physical section, or do you want to stop this journey right here?"

"What is your vision, once again, Granddaughter?" Grandfather says with a stern look.

"Well, it is the sun and the moon and the seven stars," I reply. "It's the same one it's always been, Grandfather."

"Eh, don't get testy with me, girl," he says.

"Not testy, Grandfather. Sorry," I say.

"Well, that's enough of that. Let's talk about the West section of the sacred circle known as life." He crosses his legs and sits down in front of me and Grandmother gently sits behind him. Her skirt lays out gently on the grass, covering her hand. I see her other paw lying on his shoulder. I love to see the wolf in both of them. Their human faces are wrinkled and old—their wolf faces, strong and piercing. For they are both, wolf and human. And they are more than that.

"We are thought," Grandfather says. "We are human, we are animal, we are thought, and all of that is spirit."

"Grandfather, are animals human in thought and spirit too?"

"Hmm. Everything applies for everybody, just the way it does for us. Bugs are two-legged and bugs are bugs," he says.

"Everybody has form," Grandmother says.

"It's the combination of spirit and form that makes the physical, Granddaughter," Grandfather Wolf says, waving an eagle feather back and forth. "This feather is physical, but it is pure spirit, for it is my Father Creator, Mother Creator; it is spirit, the eagle feather." It disappears and a whooshing sound spins around my ears.

"Wow, where did that feather go, Grandfather?"

"Well, it's right here, Granddaughter. Can't you see it?" and he waves it back and forth.

"I see it, Grandfather."

"Touch it, Granddaughter."

I reach out and my hand goes through all of it, the feather and him.

"You, Granddaughter, are in physical form, leaning against that pine tree. You are teaching students. We are in spirit form. We have never walked on the earth as a two-legged other than to walk as a two-legged spirit. Grandmother and I, we don't go there, we bring you here," he says.

"It was just yesterday you left here, Wolf," Grandmother Wolf says. "It was just yesterday we watched you walk off into the world of teaching. And there you are in the middle of all of it, right there."

She points, and I watch myself walk towards the teaching lodge.

"There you go."

"What am I going to tell them, Grandmother? What am I going to tell them this time?"

"Well, we're sending you to visit some really good friends of ours. In just a minute the sparkle of our leaving will be the trail to their home. Be sure to ask them, 'What am I physically?'"

I put my hand to my head and sit there in amazement. "I don't have to ask them that. I can tell you what I am. I am a worthless loser. You know, Grandfather, I failed at everything I did when I was in grade school, junior high, and high school here on the earth. I don't learn well. All my life people have been asking me to tell them the story, tell them about Mom, tell them about healing, tell them about everything. Sometimes I just want to tell them to go to..."

"Granddaughter," Grandmother says. "Don't cuss." She grins.

"Well, I like to cuss. Sometimes they ought to just go to Hell," and I laugh.

"Yeah, you like to cuss because you're ornery. You know what ornery is, Granddaughter?"

"Grandmother, sometimes, especially in the physical section of the Medicine Wheel, I don't know what anything is. The grandness of spirit overwhelms me and the mystery of physicality scares me."

"That's a good thing," Grandfather says. "Because you'll stay humble, Granddaughter. That's your job—to show humility. That's your job, to walk with the respect of humility. These friends of ours, the Bone People, they have things to say to you..."

And with that, swoosh—they were gone, and there was that twinkling, sparkling trail of stars that lingered behind them. I knew I had better move quickly, 'cause I've done this before. Those stars will be gone and I won't know where to go.

I run quickly, following the stars, moving among the trees. I run and run and run, until the trail ends in a meadow of soft yellow grass. I can hear clinking and clanging, clattering sounds all around me. Colors are swirling, swishing, twisting, spiraling and rolling, curving, and dancing around and around. As I look, the colors take form in spirit body—all spirits. As I look closer, I realize they are colored skeletons, skeletons of all kinds—four-legged, two-legged, crawly, and winged—everything that has cartilage, everything that has bone. There are thousands, no—millions and trillions—of spirit skeletons dancing!

"Oh, we're not spirit at all. You've got to get that lesson right," a voice says. "I'm a Bone Person," it growls, "and this here, she's Miz Bone."

I turn and see two Bone People standing there. Their eyes spin with color, little tiny stars fill the cavities of their eye holes, but they are pure bone. They are just like any other skeleton, a human skeleton—a two-legged with ribs and everything.

"Yep! That's us—the Bone People, at your service. Mr. Bone," and he bows, "and Mrs. Bone," she curtsies. "We're friends of your grandparents and they want us to talk to you. They want us to tell you about the bone world. You ready?" He grins a toothless grin. "You ready, you reckon? Come and follow me and I'll take you. Come on, girlfriend," and he takes his wife's hand and they dance out into the circle of exploding light.

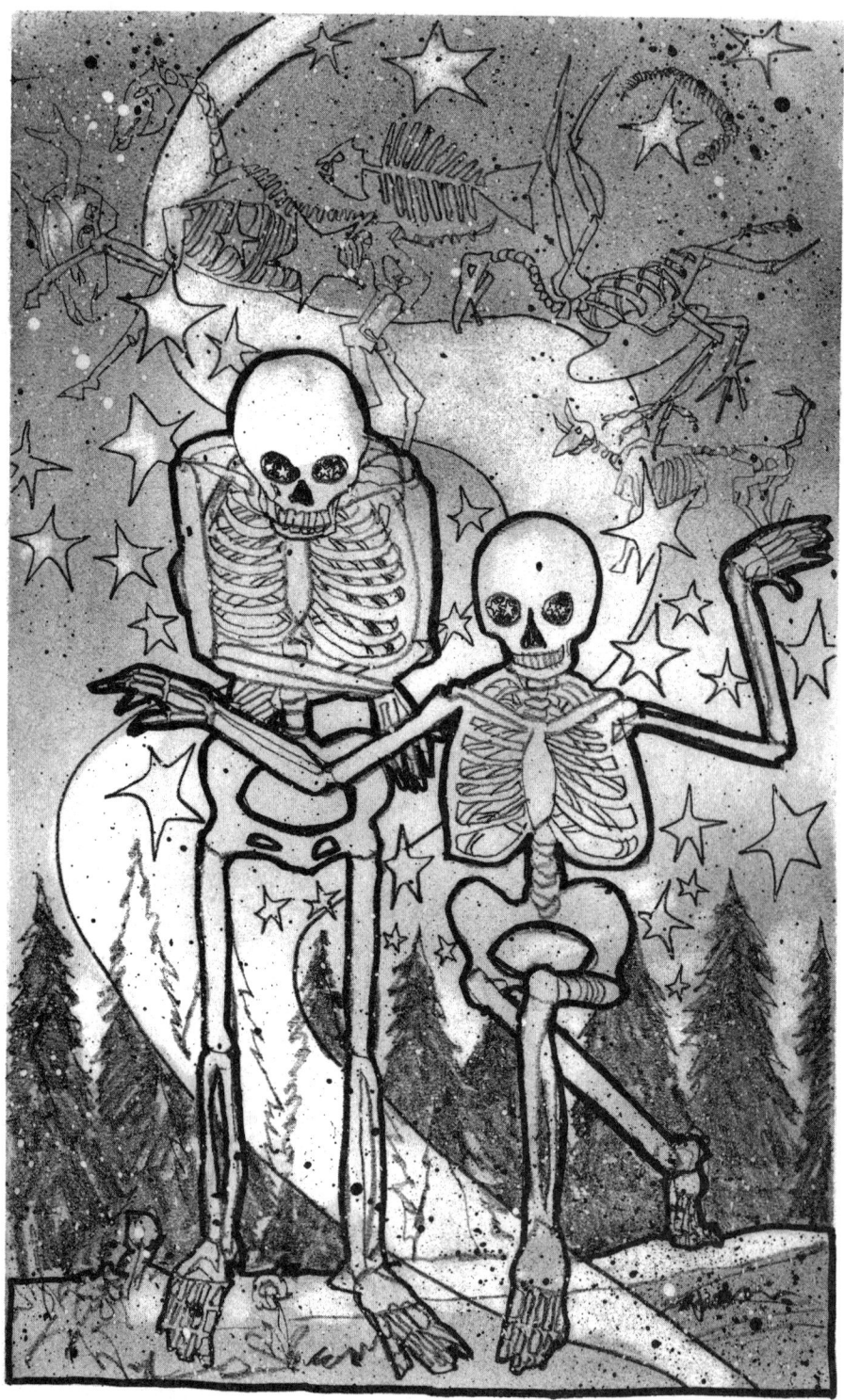

I watch them as the light explodes. Sparks fly everywhere—swirls, gases, energy, and spirit—little tiny sparks.

"Follow us," Old Bone Man shouts as they run up the hill in front of me. I take off after them. They get to the edge of the hill and stop at what is like a canyon, bigger than the Grand Canyon! Spirits fly. I see spirit people take form. In vigorous energy they burst into life.

"Now, what happens next is pure and simple development," Old Bone Man says, waving his crooked finger at me. "This mystery called life isn't that big of a deal," he says. "It's just not that big of a deal. What's the big deal is how to treat it, how to understand it, and that's where you better quit talking about yourself as being a failure, you understand?"

"Yeah," Old Bone Woman says.

"Yeah, you don't ever want to talk about yourself as a failure when you're in the physical existence. You want to see yourself as an experience," Old Bone Man says in a scratchy voice. "Now, there are a lot of things to learn about life and you're going to meet some really wise teachers. You hear me?"

Oh, I'm overcome with all those spirits. "Are they leaving to go to the Earth?"

"Earth?" he laughs. They both laugh and laugh. "Earth? That's just one small place the spirits could be going. This is the place of everything. This is the spiritual launching pad of life itself. The spirits are going to be every kind of life that has bone. You know, there are other places you can go, too. You can see how the plant people come and you can see how the water people start. All you've got to do is follow that path over there."

I see a spiraling path of color.

"Everything starts here. Right here. You know, some say this is the face of God, right here," and he laughs.

"Well, how did I get to be here?"

"How did you get to be here?" he says with a puzzled look on his face. "How did you get to be here? Well, your Grandmother and Grandfather Wolf sent you here, and I'm sure you're on your own adventure. Don't use up my time now, girl, I've got to tell you this," and he takes his little walking stick and starts moving. And there they go, these rattling, clanking, clanging sets of bones holding hands, heading off.

I think that's my invitation to follow, and I strike out after them, running with all four feet on the ground—here comes the Wolf, tongue hanging out, two legs moving one in front of the other.

"Wait! Wait!"

"Yeah, you'd better say wait. You'll never understand anything about the sacred circle if you can't comprehend physical existence. Ho, ho, ho," he laughs.

They stop dead still, and a wave of sound—bigger than huge—comes over me.

"What is that?" It's like millions of people singing at one time. It's like the most beautiful sound that has ever, ever been in my head.

"Well, that," Old Bone Man says softly, "is the voice of Big Music," and he bows his head.

Old Bone Woman bows her head. "Bow your head," she whispers to me.

I bow my head.

"That's right. We told you to do it, because it is sacred to bow your head to the Big Music. That's the Voice of God. That's the Voice of Creator. Here in the Face is the Voice."

With my head still bowed, I listen to the singing. The sounds are the color blue. They actually sound blue, the sound of deep tranquility.

"Yep. All color has sound. All sound has color," Old Bone Woman says.

I can hear rattling. Rattles, drums and dancers. I can see color—spirals and points of light.

"There is a spirit getting ready to take form right in front of your face," Old Bone Man says, sticking his finger out. "The Big Music calls form into motion."

The spiraling color grows large, very large. Huge it is.

"What is that?"

"Oh, that? That's Big Music taking form. You'll see him. You'll meet him."

"Can I ask a question?" I say to Old Bone Man, as we raise our heads.

"Yeah. Yeah, you can," Old Bone Man says.

"How come we have to die? How come we have to get sick? And how come I can't get..."

"Shh," Old Bone Woman says. "I know that thought you are thinking and the answer to it is, it is not your job to get other people to do things. It is your job to tell them the Truth. Spiritual medicine is Truth," she says, shaking her cane at me.

"The answers to your questions are right ahead of you, on this Red Road you are following."

"The Red Road is the voice of spirit, you know," Old Bone Man says. "And you need to understand that we're going to talk about the physical road, and that's the Blue Road. The blue—that's the West. You've got to listen to that. In your vision, in your Rainbow Medicine Wheel, that blue gate is the doorway to the physical road. The body and the mind are the Blue Road. You come to it by following the Red Road till you get to the end and the blue gate becomes the Blue Road. Now, are you confused?" he says with a laugh.

"Well, sometimes this medicine work is hard. It's hard to tell the Blue Road from the Red Road." I say. "I have learned that the Red Road is a long, good road of the spirit, and the Blue Road is the road of physicality that ends in death. So that makes the Blue Road a road that isn't a circle, but the Red Road is probably a circle. That is, if the Red Road is the only real road and everything—"

"Oh, man! You human beings! You get to thinking so fast you can't even keep up with a concept," Old Bone Woman says. "It doesn't matter. When you're teaching these people, it's a circle with two lines—one going up and down and one going from side to side." She leans over, takes her finger and draws in the dirt. "It's a symbol lying flat, so they can see the Red Road and they can see the Blue Road, but you start the Red Road in physical existence at the beginning, in the East. You come in through the spirit and you walk up to the body. Now, you can go around and come to the body—you just walk in through the East gate and make that arch around through the medicines."

"You got that?" Old Bone Man looks at me. "Or you can go right straight up, and you'll be at the West gate like you came in to see us today. You got that? You see, the symbol is the wheel on the ground, and you look inside the gate into the school of spirit, which is where you are now. Now you get that all figured out, then you'll understand how those little tiny spirits right there are going to come into life. They're going to drop right into the form of a physical being—their mother, the moon," he says. "You know, the moon?"

"They're going to drop into the moon?" I ask.

"No, no, no, no." Old Bone Man puts his hand to his head and says,

"I haven't got time to say this. Your chapter's going to be up pretty soon and they're going to read this one of these days and think I don't know anything, and it's just because you're taking up all my time! Remember, you're writing a book! Remember, you're teaching. Remember that you came here to listen to us. You came to us because of your vision that you had when you were little, because we gave it to you from your Grandfather and your Grandmother Wolf. Have you got it?" He points his walking stick right at my heart. "That's right, I'm a-pointing at you. You've got to remember everything. Anyhow, they're going to come into their mother. The moon medicine. Moon. Woman. Right?"

Old Bone Woman says, "Woman medicine. Listen. Woman! Moon!" and she starts waving her finger around, pointing up and down, and going, "The moon! Right? Okay! The father is the sun," she says, "and the mother is the moon, and they got together and all these stars burst out from everywhere. That's Creation. That's God. That's the Circle of Creation. That's Great Spirit's holiness emerging into school, which is Real, and Real is a medicine. When you understand Real, then you've got to understand your Grand, girl."

"I'm Grand," I say. "No—I'm lost, I'm not Grand. Are you trying to tell me that I'm Grand? Are you trying to tell me how those spirit things out there are going somewhere? I'm lost."

"You're not lost," Old Bone Man says. "You're just like any other two-legged, you just don't want to listen. So there! I've had enough of it. Listen for the rattling and the clicking. If you ain't a-listening, then you ain't going to know," he says.

"Can I ask you one more question?"

"You'd better hurry." He's starting to get up off the ground.

"Are you going to go down and go to a mother and become an existence? Is that what you were trying to tell me? Are you trying to tell me that those swirling lights become a bone, and then they become a human?"

"No. They're a human when they're a bone, I'm a-saying. I'm a human. I'm a Bone."

"You can't be," I say. "We're in the spirit world."

"No, no, no. We're not in the spirit world. You're in the spirit world looking at us. We *are* spirit."

"I thought you said you were a human." I look at him through my hair hanging down in my eyes. Poof—I blow it up off my forehead.

"You're making it a lot harder than it is, and how are you going to answer their questions about life and death if you don't even understand it yourself? You're going to walk in there in just a minute and tell them people you know everything."

He is gone. She is gone. And I am saying "Aho."

I come to the end of my prayer that evening and open my eyes to the seven new students who sit before me in the circle. He is right. It's my job now to teach the West section of the Rainbow Medicine Wheel, which is the physical section, as I teach it.

"Well, who am I?" I say, and I lean back and put my head against the wall. "Who am I to tell you what anything is, and that's what I want to start with tonight. Everything is an opinion. Everybody has one—they're like butt holes." I have some smiles and some laughter, and some people look at me like "Huh?" I know exactly how they feel, because I don't have the answers. "I'm going to tell you that right out. That life and death is a mystery. It's an unknown."

One student looks at me and says, "I didn't come here not to get my questions answered, so you're sure not going to tell me that there are no answers to life and death, are you?"

"Oh, no. I have no intention of telling you that."

I hear the rattling of the bones calling me back.

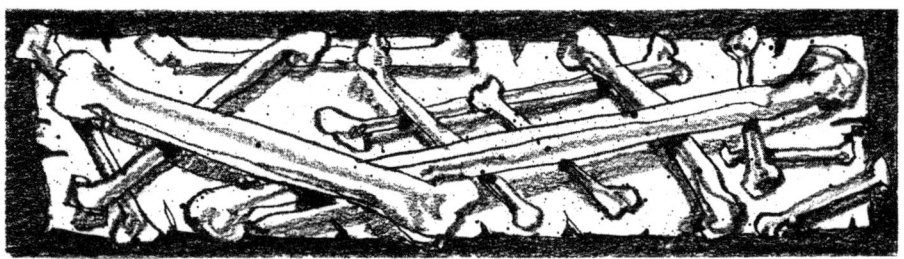

Personal Journal

When you are studying Bone Medicine, I recommend that you keep a personal journal. In it you will record all your feelings while you are reading the words in this book. I recommend that you keep this personal journal for life—for your entire physical existence. It is a good way to keep your feelings in order, a good way to look back and remember what you did. Personal journals are meant to emphasize what is personal in your life. They are not for anyone else. You can share them with someone else, if you choose to, but never let anyone read your journal, and no one should ever want to read your journal without your permission.

A journal can be any size. I recommend a spiral notebook or a 5 x 7 notebook—small enough to go anywhere and big enough to record everything. Once you have filled up one journal, start a new one. Keep the journals organized and dated, so you can file them in an appropriate order, so that when you're looking for something, it's easy to pull it out.

You will find that, in the exercises and ceremonies in the book, there are times I will ask you to record your thoughts in your journal. This will help you to get started journaling. I have used a journal since I was six years old and it is very valuable to me, for I have many, many experiences. By keeping a personal journal, I have the ability to tell myself the truth about what really happened.

There are all types of journals—video recorded ones, computer based ones, tape recorded ones—these are all good—whatever you choose in the modern world. In the old way, they were pictographs.

Aho.

Physical Medicine Teachings

The West section of the Rainbow Medicine Wheel is the physical section. Physical is matter. It is solid. It houses our existence, which is our thought, spirit, and emotions. A Rainbow Medicine Wheel is like any other medicine wheel or ancient teaching of a medicine wheel—the spirit, the emotions, the body, and the mind.

Long ago and now come together when you work with a medicine wheel. It is spiritual, for it is not provable. No one can ever prove or disprove life. As hard as we try to make the physical concrete, it has other components. Within the Rainbow Medicine Wheel, in the West section, the teachings are of the Fall, the teachings of maturity, the teachings of the body, of the physical—defined as bodily, fleshly, earthly, visible, solid, actual, existence.

There are seven medicine stones within the Rainbow Medicine

Wheel's West section of physicality. Those seven stones are the medicines that you apply to your life. From my vision I have learned that the seven stars in the West section are known as red—Nurture, orange—Choice, yellow—Ceremony, green—Change, blue—Proof, purple—Real, burgundy—Grand.

There are seven physical lesson stones. They are red—purpose; orange—obedience; yellow—life; green—action; blue—solid; purple—full; burgundy—worthy. In defining physicality I have connected Nurture to bodily, Choice to fleshly; Ceremony to earthly; Change to visible; Proof to solid; Real to actual; and Grand to existence. By doing this I am saying that the seven medicine stones, with the words I have connected to them, are understandings that will help you deal with your lessons. The medicine stone words treat your physicality in a way where you can see that bodily is vital. Bone is form—it is a body; it is vital, it is living. Fleshly is mass—blood, cells, and dying. Earthly is cycles—it is death and decay; it is Fall; it is West. Visible is vision—it is color; it is spirit. Solid is material—it is concrete; it is matter. Actual is real—it is concrete; it is definition; it is truth. Existence is essential—it is spirit; it is beliefs; it is thought.

These words that I share with you are the circle of physicality. When we apply our seven medicine words to our physicality and live with Nurturing, live with our fleshly Choices, live with our earthly Ceremonies, live with our visible Changes, live with our solid Proof, live with our actual Real, live with our Grandness in existence—we are living our physical medicine teachings. As humans, we will experience sickness and death. But each of us has choices with which we can change our sickness or death.

We can get a clear understanding that our cells hold within them the story of life. All we have to do is ask and remember that our DNA gives us our unique structure of personality and character, that we have blood, tissue, muscle, fat, water, hair, skin, teeth, eyeballs, and vessels—that we are made up of a complex symphony of vibration, sound, and color. Within the physical medicine teachings, look at yourself as a sacred circle—you are unique only to yourself. Self is your specialness. Each physical being is a human; we are all human. We breathe, we reproduce, we eat, we die. We don't understand that individualism is the self—the personality. And only if it has character is personality individual. Each human is the same human; there are two kinds—male and female. When you are physical, you learn you are not unique unless you have the whole self, which is to have an awakened spirit. Then you have self. Our spirit is our code to uniqueness. It is our pattern to individuality.

Aho.

Medicine Blanket

A medicine blanket may start by a mother making it. A lot of us don't have a mother, though, who would make us one. And a lot of people get detached from their medicine blanket even when their mother did make one for them. That's what stores are for, so go and get a new one. The blanket can be anything—it can be handmade; it can be a quilt; it can be a tapestry of any type. It can be old pieces of blankets sewn together that have been your mother's, and her mother's. It can be cloth that comes from shirts that have been in the family for a long time. The cloth becomes a blanket, and the blanket becomes a medicine blanket, because it has you in it—your oils, your smells, your actions, your memories. The blanket is yours.

I recommend the Pendelton wool blanket for a good medicine blanket, or a 100% cotton serape from Mexico.

I have seen many, many sacred medicine blankets. I was given mine at a young age and I have carried it through everything and have it today. It is an adult, mature blanket, for it is twenty-four years old now. It has walked with me for a long time. It will be the blanket that I am wrapped and buried in.

Your medicine blanket is personal to you, but you do have the choice of passing it on at any time to someone else, to give someone else security with it. It is a transitional tool that helps you deal with being scared, alone, frightened, or angry. I suggest that you use your medicine blanket, and it will comfort you. Wrap it around you to draw in your inner strength and power. Carry it to shelter you, to protect you, to give you warmth and sacredness. Sleep under it, cling to it, pray with it, fold it, and place it in a sacred way.

A medicine blanket is always with you.

Aho.

Making Prayer Ties

The term "making prayers" is one I would like to share. A prayer tie enables you to "make" a prayer. To make a prayer, you take a piece of cloth or paper, put a pinch of tobacco or herb in it, gather it together, wrap it with a string, tie it, and string it on a prayer line, along with others. Then you move on and make another prayer tie that you tie to the same line. One prayer tie equals one prayer.

After we finish making prayer ties, and have strung them all on a line, we wrap the line and the string of prayers around a stick and carry it to the Medicine Wheel. There it is unwrapped, and the "prayers" are either laid in the center of the wheel or hung on prayer lines that circle the Medicine Wheel.

When I learned about prayer ties, I was taught that a fat prayer tie is a fat prayer, and a fat prayer contains a lot of thought. As I got older, I began to realize that applied to people, too. I don't see fat as sickness; I see it as a lot of thought. I see it as a large happening. When I see a whale, I see a large prayer tie. When I see a little teeny, tiny baby—I see a teeny, tiny prayer.

Making prayer ties can be done as often as needed. I suggest sunrise, noon, evening, and midnight. A prayer tie is a prayer in physical form, and praying in thought is making prayer in a spiritual form. I believe that you can be in constant prayer, for your thoughts—every one of them—can be constant, reverent, beautiful action.

When you go to make a prayer tie, the color of cloth or paper you use will represent the medicines or the lessons that you are working with in the prayer. Sometimes I tie a double prayer tie onto the line, representing the color for the lesson I am working with, and the color of the medicine I am applying to my life to bring forth the outcome that I wish. And sometimes when I make prayer, I make two actual prayer ties—one for the lesson and one for the medicine.

Below is an example of a prayer tie.

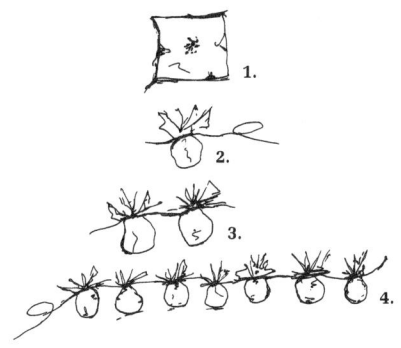

It is a good thing to make at least one prayer tie every day. We can make four prayers to represent the four directions every day, or we can make seven prayers, one for each color of each medicine and each lesson that we live. Or we can tie an unlimited number of prayer ties to represent a large, large prayer. Our choice of making prayer is up to us as individuals. When we hang our prayer ties on the lines or put them in the center of the wheel, this represents letting go of the prayer and letting it return to Grandmother/Grandfather. On each solstice of the year, I gather the prayer ties and burn them, which represents the final dismissal of the physical prayer tie, allowing the prayer to be carried away in the smoke to Great Spirit.

It is important to remember that your prayer is heard at the moment it is prayed, and that making and having the physical prayer tie hung, or lying in the center of the wheel, is an action of respect, a symbol of prayer in physical form, and your understanding at the time you prayed it. Then you carry it to the solstice and dismiss it. When you have a physical form of prayer, such as a prayer tie, it represents the physical body, and it is a good thing to change the physical form into spirit. This is done when you dismiss the prayer by burning it.

In the old ways, there were lots of prayers—for hunting, gathering, marriage, family, sickness, death, birth. Keep this in mind when you set your intention in doing prayers.

Aho.

Ceremony of the Sacred Herbs

The Ceremony of the Sacred Herbs is often called smudging. Smudging is done by gathering an herb and burning it. Often the herbs are called medicines. I recommend that you use an all-natural bowl made from stone or some other nonflammable material—an abalone shell is good.

You also need a fan, which can be one feather or several feathers bound together, or you can use your hand to wave across the smoke from the herb when it is burning.

The Ceremony of the Sacred Herbs is used for balancing and cleansing the air, balancing negative and positive ions. It can be used to lift your spirits and make you feel good, for the sweet smells of the herbs are wonderful and uplifting. I recommend that you do the smudging ceremony with sweet grass, sage, piñon, cedar, or juniper. The ones that are most commonly used are sage and sweet grass. You can locate these herbs at various supply stores, such as trading posts, bead stores, herb stores, and health food stores, or you can go and gather them on your own from the cedar tree, the juniper tree, or the sage bush. Be sure to leave tobacco or a pinch of cornmeal or a song or whistle—something to give back for their gift to you.

There are other sacred herbs that you can burn, and the Ceremony of the Sacred Herbs is often called "burning incense."

The ceremony starts with lighting the herbs and placing them in the bowl. Then you fan across the bowl, moving the smoke in a circular motion to cleanse the energy field around your body to help bring balance and calm to your physical existence. It is important to remember to move the sage bowl or the herb, allowing the smoke to travel all around your body, back and front, under your feet and above your head. At the end of the ceremony, reach out your hand and pull it through the smoke to your heart to honor the sacredness of the smoke and the sacredness of Great Spirit.

I do not recommend that any banishing herb or drug, such as marijuana, tobacco, juniper, frankincense, or myrrh, be used in this ceremony. Select only herbs that bring about a positive uplifting and are known as healing herbs.

When you are finished, extinguish the burning herbs, and put your fan and bowl away by placing them on your altar or in a sacred place. Aho.

How to Build a Rainbow Medicine Wheel

The Rainbow Medicine Wheel is a circle built of 68 stones. It is a sacred site meant to be a place of prayer and self study. Each rock has a meaning. There are four directions in the Rainbow Medicine Wheel, one of spirit, one of emotion, one of the physical body, which is the place of Bone Medicine, and one of the mind. In each one of these sections, there are seven medicine stones and seven lesson stones. The center of the wheel represents the seven sacred stars and Great Spirit, Creator, God.

When you build a Rainbow Medicine Wheel, select a special place in your home or outdoors on your property. Use your favorite stones of red, orange, yellow, green, blue, purple, and burgundy. The stones can be of any size; I recommend large ones for a large medicine wheel, small ones for an indoor medicine wheel.

It is important that the medicine wheel be placed where it is private and will be honored. No loud noise, anger, drugs, or alcohol is to be present. Place it where animals and children will not run through it. When you need a place to study, pray, or perform a ceremony, the medicine wheel is there for you. It is a place to go when you are in grief, loneliness, or joy, and wanting to speak with Great Spirit.

The Rainbow Medicine Wheel is what I like to call a rock church/school. For a long time Natives have gathered at the rock

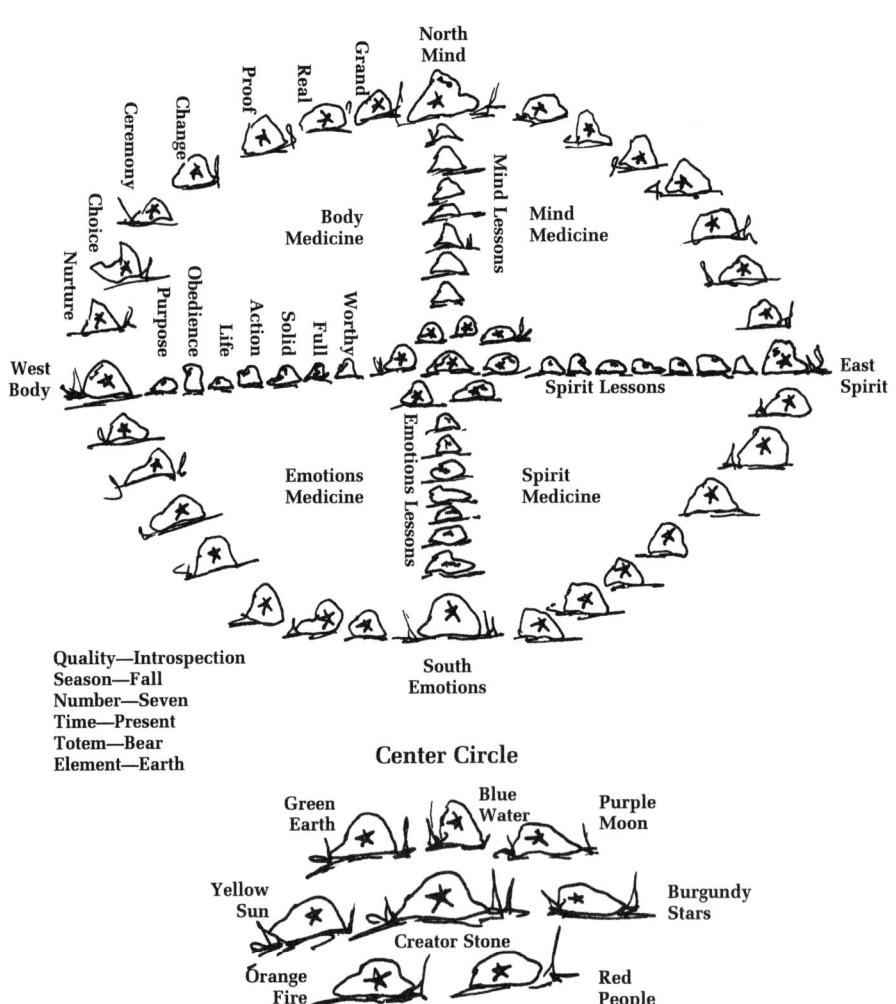

Rainbow Medicine Wheel

church to hold sacred ceremonies such as weddings, funerals, namings, and rites of passage. Today we use it to sit and do our journaling and shamanic journeys to connect with the spirit world, as well as perform sacred ceremonies. It is to be a place of comfort and joy.

When building a medicine wheel, you start by smudging the area and yourself. The size you build your medicine wheel depends on how many people you want to have around it in a circle. It is important to find the center spot and start there with your Creator stone (see the illustration).

Before you place the stones, offer a giveaway to the center spot and a prayer to Great Spirit for each stone that will be placed. In your mind, envision a spiral. Start with the center stone, and, moving outward, place your second stone on the right-hand side of the center. Continue placing stones until you have completed the center circle.

Moving outward to the direction stones, place the east stone on the right-hand side, the south stone at the bottom, the west stone to the left and the north stone at the top.

Standing at the East stone, now place the lesson stones—red, orange, yellow, green, blue, purple, and burgundy—in a straight line in each section towards the center. Standing at the East stone, place the seven medicine stones so that they make a circle, completing the medicine wheel.

There are no rules at the Rainbow Medicine Wheel. There is just the right way, which is moving clockwise. It is a must, to bring forth a good Red Road, that you move always in a clockwise direction. When you move counterclockwise, you are walking the Blue Road, which is physical existence and therefore an end, death, and dismissal; and lessons come to you.

The Rainbow Medicine Wheel honors all people, all beliefs, all lessons. It is a visible connection to the Sacred Hoop of Life—oneself.

You are the keeper of your medicine wheel. You may keep it as long as you wish, and are using it. If you should decide to change locations, or that you no longer wish to study at a Rainbow Medicine Wheel, or you would just simply like to take it down and rebuild it, do so by starting with the last stone and going through the ceremony backwards. Finish the process by smudging yourself and the area in which the wheel has been placed.

Medicine wheels are constructed by medicine teachers. This medicine wheel is mine to give you from my vision of the sun, the moon, and the seven stars. There are many medicine wheels; there are complicated ways to place one, and there are simple ways. A medicine wheel can have spirit poles that form the gateways and the skeletal structure of a medicine wheel, as well as spirit cords that protect and surround the medicine wheel area. In *Bone Medicine*, I use the simple wheel, for I like to think of physicality as simple. I feel that you will enjoy the energy of a medicine wheel and learn many lessons from its existence. Remember that it is flow, and we must never fight the flow of lessons.

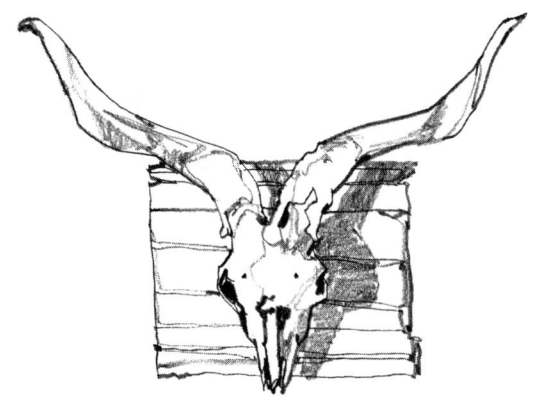

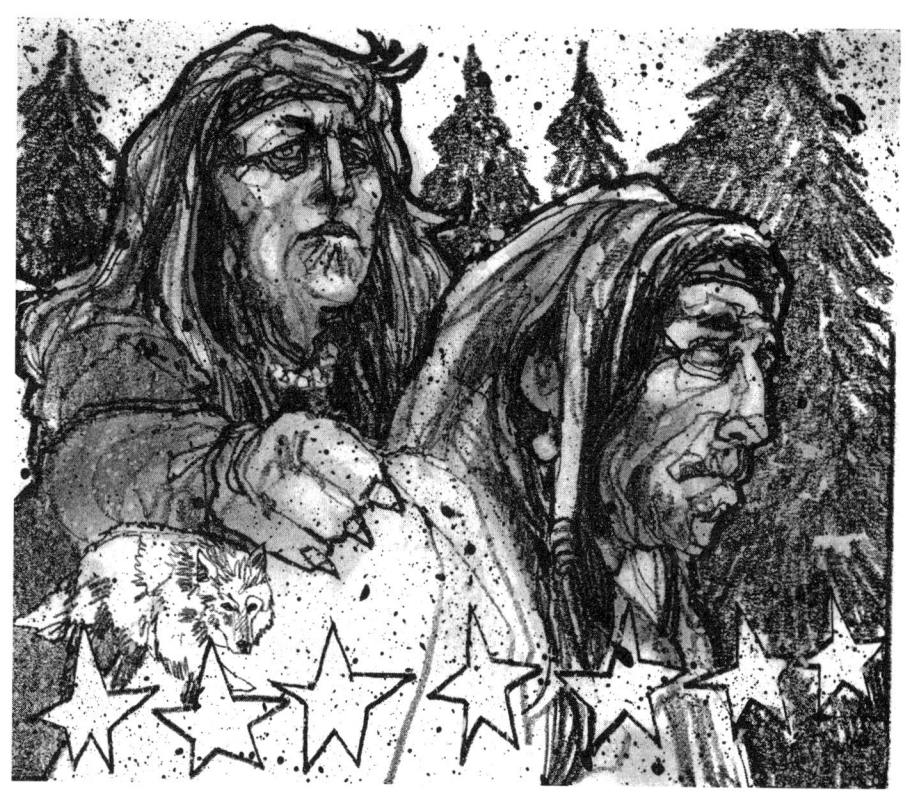

2
THE GATEWAY OF THE WEST

(CIRCLE OF THE BEAR)

Before me I see two poles forming a gate; a blue flag is blowing in the breeze. I watch the cloth gently sway backwards and forwards. The sun is setting; the quiet evening has come. Darkness is falling. The smells of autumn fill my mind—fireplaces burning, wet leaves, and fresh earth. I take a deep breath and blow out the cool evening air and watch my breath and the smoke dancing, leaving me.

I breathe in, I sniff—it's a funny smell. Yuck, it stinks. The fresh aroma of wet leaves becomes decay. A dead smell—moldy, rotten. Yuck! Just pure stink. I hear a low rumbling sound behind me in the trees. Fear sets in around me. The hair on the back of my neck is rising up. I turn and look into the trees. I can tell a presence is there, and I start walking that way. Then in front of me are footprints—enormous footprints, similar to a human's—probably a size 15 to 17 shoe, but there are scratch marks at the top of the footprints. Hmm. I stop, frozen, knowing that these are bear tracks.

A loud roar rings out, growling sounds and the breaking of limbs. It is all around me—I feel my heart pounding. The smells become more intense, and I feel breathing next to me. I take a breath and force myself to look. In all four directions around me stand figures—enormous figures—with intense feelings. Their eyes are looking straight at me. I am confronted and encircled by four bears. To the East of me is a brown bear, with beady black eyes. In the South there is a black bear, with a band of tan masking its face. Its eyes are black and beady too, and it is huge as it stands on all four paws, looking at me quietly. I look to the West and there is a gigantic bear with long, long nails. It is standing on its two hind feet. It opens its mouth and roars, a beastly groan. Its teeth are fang-like. It is a grizzly, over thirteen feet tall. I look to the North and there is a polar bear, standing up on its huge hind legs.

The bears growl, and the vibration of the sound shatters the air around me. I grab my ears and drop to the ground, as the bears start to walk towards me. My mind shuts down in total fear. A mist of darkness comes over me, blue and purple, white, black, and silver. I am lying on my back, looking into the faces of all four. The grizzly has pushed me backwards and now has its right front paw on my chest. It kneels down. I am looking into the eyes of a man—a two-legged with the features of a bear. Strong nose, piercing black eyes, strong in stature and dark in color, he has golden, honey-colored skin. He is bare to the waist.

"Thank you for joining us, Wolf," he says in a deep, piercing voice. "I am Big Music. I speak with the voice of Great Spirit. I am Grizzly Bear, the first keeper of the Creator's form. I have taken form in the blue night sky, far beyond this place. I am no longer earthly. I am not bound to Earth. I am the mature form of the West—a mature male. These are my relatives. The small brown bear, there across from me, is the spirit of the West. He is known as Soft Spirit. That one in the South, the black

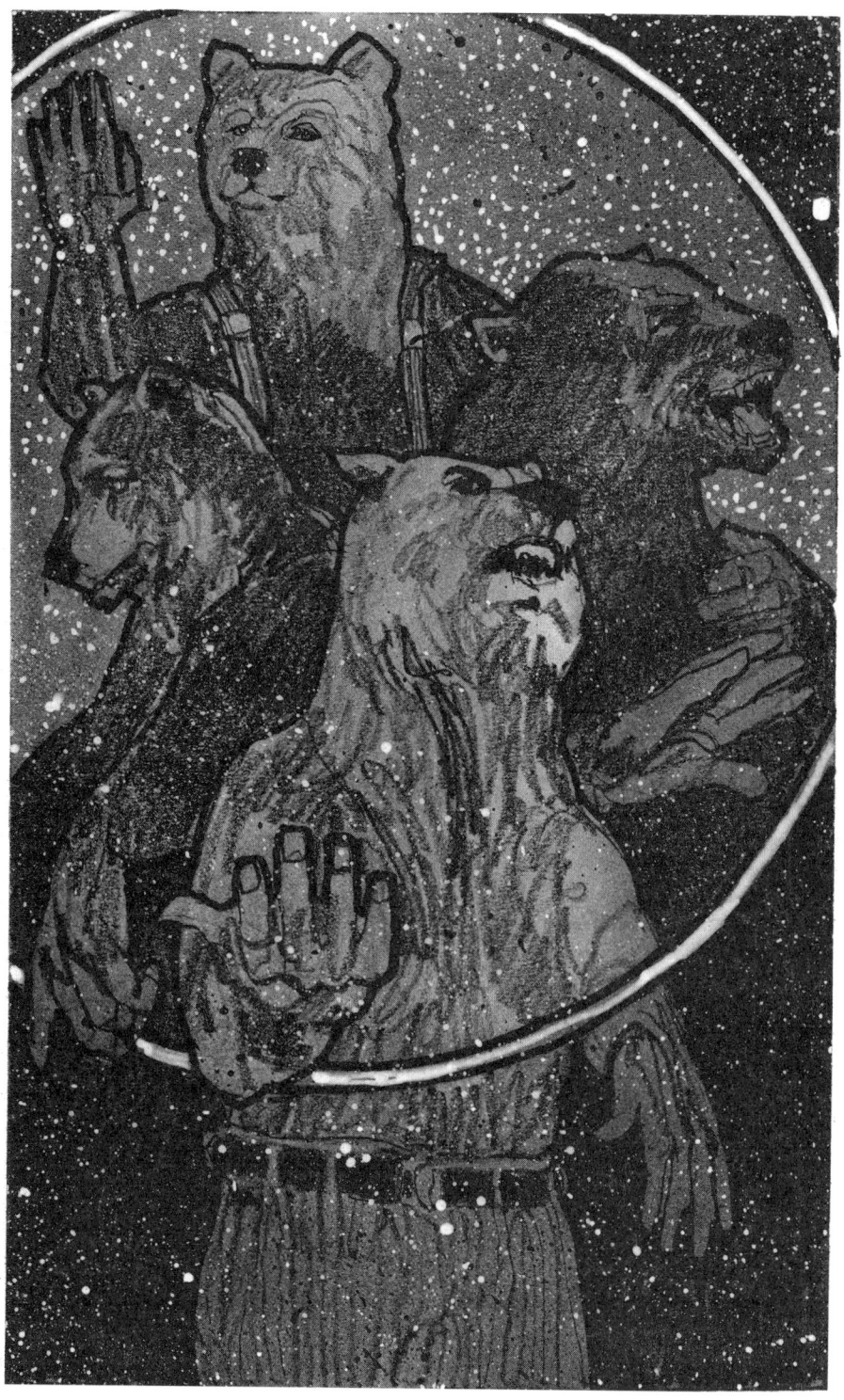

one, is known as Standing Bear. And in the North, that white one is known as the North Wind. We are the Sacred Circle of the Council of Bear Medicine. We are the family of the bear. In the four-legged clan we are the Bear People, the Bear Clan. In your world we walk as bear and man. Our family knows no difference between the two-legged and the four-legged, for as you see, we stand on two legs."

I look up, and he stands above me, a huge, mature, Native American male. Beside him stand an elder, a Native American man with long white hair, a very young Native American child, and a teenaged Native American male.

"I am showing you the four levels of the West. I am the directional guide, keeper, overseer," he says. "Remember, I am Big Music."

I sit up, shake my head a little, and realize that I am in the teachings of the West.

"Which one of you is Death?" I ask. "Which one of you is sickness? I think you must be birth," and I look at the young one. He is making silly faces at me, sticking his tongue out, and wiggling his ears.

Big Music sits down cross-legged in front of me. He picks up some twigs and stacks them like a teepee. He pulls some grass from the ground, lays it in the center of the twig teepee, and lights a small fire. He starts putting some little sticks on it, and before long it is a comfortable, quiet fire. There is a suspended feeling all around us and if I move to the right or to the left, I feel dizzy. So I just sit, very focused and very quiet. I look Big Music in the face, deep into his dark eyes.

"Where is death?"

Big Music looks at me sternly. "Right there," he says, pointing to my heart. "Right there, in you. For it is time. It is the place. That's not what you have come here for, though. It is mine to see that you understand that the West is Introspection, that you have to understand inside," and he places his hand on his heart. "Inside, Wolf, is Introspection. You must be like a turtle and pull your head deep down inside yourself, to know Introspection."

"Which one of you is Introspection?" I ask.

"We are all the West. We are the four movements within the circle of the West." He moves his hand in a spiraling motion and pulls the other three into a swirling, spinning mist of white and black color, which he draws into his hand, and sucks through his mouth noisily. Then he lifts his chin and says, "It is all me. I am the West. I am the overseer of the physical existence. Everything answers to me, in Introspection, in knowing the self. These students and you, and every two-legged who exists, want to know why we are human."

"I didn't realize that I came here to find out why I'm human. I didn't remember even thinking that."

He laughs with a deep voice. "You've always wondered why."

"Yeah. Yeah, I have. And I'll tell you something, if you're in charge of human, I've got a few bones to pick with you," I say, getting up slowly and standing above him. I'm feeling quite proud of myself, looking down on Big Music.

In the twinkling of an eye he is standing tall above me, and looking down at me. He says, "Well," smacking his lips, "Have you ever seen a bear and a wolf tangle?"

"Yeah. Yeah, I—I saw it on TV, and the wolf actually won," I say, feeling quite proud of myself. I can actually feel my tail swishing back and forth. "Yeah. Yeah, I can take you on."

"Ha, ha, ha," he laughs. His eyes are wild and full of fire. "Take me on—let's see...Intentions. What are your intentions? That's the only way I want to take you on."

"Well, my intentions are the bones that I have to pick with you. I want you to understand that I'm not too happy with the fact that, that, well—" I kind of hesitate and stammer a little bit. "I'll tell you, if you're in charge of death or know anything about why people get sick or why people hurt innocent people, I—I'm really looking forward to—to—to—uh—having the answers," I stutter.

"Just a little afraid of the answers, are you, Wolf?" he says. "That's usually what human beings do, is they pick a fight and then they stammer around, and then they get one punch and it's over. The ground is made up of a bunch of dead beings that tried to find the answers and fell by the wayside."

"I don't want to be one of those people, Big Music. I want to know more about life coming into form. The old Bone Woman and the old Bone Man, they showed me something I need to remember."

"Yes, they did, Wolf," he says scratching his cheek. "They showed you something very, very powerful about color. Walk with me," and he turns and starts walking into the woods. "Soon I will be a polar bear, and then I will be a bone man, and then I will be pure sound. You understand?"

I stop and look at him carefully. "I want to understand, and I want to teach, and I want to know. But I have to tell you something. There are two things in life that are really hard for me right now, and that's a set of dark eyes. Someone I hold dear." I drop my head, and breathe slowly. "Why is it, Big Music, we have to have sadness in our lives. Why can't we get what we want? That's a good question—do you have an answer for that? How come we make mistakes? How come we, as two-leggeds, are so inadequate? Is somebody mad at us?" I turn and look deep into the woods. There is a quiet that stabilizes me inside.

"Oh, Wolf. Do people ask you all of this?"

"YES!" I said sternly. "Yes, they do. Constantly. They want a good life. They want enough money, they want enough time, they want enough children, they want to be loose from their children, they want to get over their mistakes, they want to make mistakes. You know?"

He stops me with his paw/hand on my shoulder, and says, "Who signed up for the job? Who was it, when her sister was dying, demanded an answer? Who was it, when she was a young child of seven, losing her caregiver, demanded an answer?"

"Yeah, and I still demand that answer," I say quickly. "I demand an answer for sickness and for death. Introspection is your answer, I'm sure. I need to go inside and find the answer. It's always inside and it's always me doing all the work. I don't want to do the work. I want someone to tell me. This is the spirit world, aren't I right?"

"Well, this is a mixture," he says. "This is a mixture of spirit and physical, for you are real and I am real. I am the keeper of the West. I can teach you bodily things. I can teach you earthly things. I can tell you about maturity. I can tell you about the Fall. I can allow you to walk towards the North within my knowledge and I can share with you that death is a great doorway."

"Is death a bear?" I ask. "Is that all there is to it, a mighty swing of a bear's paw and it's all over? If that's the case, then why do we bother in the first place? That's the thing my students are always asking me, and that's what I want to know."

"Heh, heh," he laughs, kneeling down. "You see, everyone tries to make life what they want it to be and everyone wants the answers. I'm not the answers. I am the keeper of the West. Do you know what that means?" he asks.

"You oversee it, right? You take care of it," I say.

"Yes, I do. I am in charge of the physical existence. The physical part of the Red Road is mine, to see it become a reality—which is the Blue Road. There are only two roads in life—a spiritual road and a physical road. Everyone is always concerned about death, dying, and sickness, because they don't understand that it's all a circle," he says, with his hands extended, two fingers pointing out. "Life is opportunity. It is a chance to hear, to feel, and to live the Big Music. I *am* the keeper of physicality," and he crosses his arms on his chest. "Wolf, we could talk all night and all day, and I will be here for you, and I will show you."

The air is still and quiet. I am overcome with questions and thoughts, the journals of my students, pain.

"All I know, Big Music, is death never has felt good to me. Up ahead of me, is death for my mom? Is death for me? Is death for my half-side?"

"Tsk, tsk, Wolf. It's deeper than that. All you have to do is set the intention and remember Introspection," and his voice echoes away, deep in my mind. "Introspection...introspection...introspection..."

I hear the rattling of the bones calling me back.

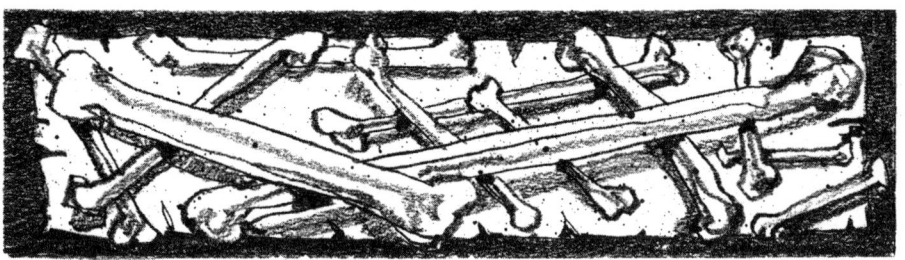

Ceremony of Introspection

TOOLS: *White candle; pen and journal; medicine blanket; two-foot (60cm) long stick; blue cotton cloth that is 24 inches long by 2 inches wide (60cm x 5cm), cut in strips; a quiet place to perform the ceremony; smudge bowl, feather, and herbs.*

The Ceremony of Introspection gives you a chance to get in touch with yourself and to record these feelings in your journal so that you can draw from your inner strengths, and expand your confidence and self-esteem.

Introspection is the depth of your physical outreach in life. By that I mean you are self—you are a total medicine—you are a circle of energy. Before you do anything, before you go out into the world, your clans and your mother, your grandmother, your father, and grandfather, aunts, and uncles should teach you the seven movements that show you the inner way to look at things. I have listed a few questions that you can ask yourself to help with that.

The movements of introspection are:

1. Examination. To look at yourself and at what you want to do.

2. Analysis. This means to take everything apart, to look at what's behind everything.
Example: You need money in order to live. Make a list of what you need money for, and then figure out how many hours you'll have to work to get it.

This is taking apart—analyzing why you need money in your life.

3. Heart searching. This takes place when you expand your feelings into what you want to do.
Example: Boy, I wish there was an easier way to make money to take care of myself, so I think I'll find something to do in life I really enjoy.

4. Counsel. This is to question your reasoning—looking at both sides of the physical reason to have money—or any other matter at hand.
Example: Well, what does it matter if it's not easy to make money? I'm still going to need the money to survive. No, I think I can pick something I like to do and, therefore, I'll enjoy what I do to make my money.

5. Deliberation. Here you run your plan through your mind and listen to your reasoning. This is actually a deep counseling during which you continue to argue and state the opinions and the facts that oppose you in what you want to do.
Example: Well, it doesn't matter if it's easy or if it's not easy. I don't like to work. Well, I have to work, I don't have any choice. I don't get money unless I work. Well, I'll probably fail at it because I don't like to do anything—I'm lazy. No, I'm not lazy.

I just don't like to do things for work that I don't enjoy.

6. Reflection. Reflection is thought, just generally easy thought.
Example: Well, work is hard. Yeah, but I've got to have money. Well, there are probably a lot of ways to make money, so I need to find the right one. Which one is that? Well, it will have to be something I like. No, not always. There are things I can do that I don't like. Yeah, well, I've worked before and the things that I seem to do successfully are the things I like to do.

7. Soul Searching. Soul searching is listening to your inner thoughts, and that means reaching into your creativity and into your potential.
Example: I think the reason that I want to do what I want to do when I work is because it is connected to helping other people. I am very clear that the purpose of work is to help other people. No other reason.

Introspection takes you in a free-flowing circle in which you can take everything apart and analyze, counsel, deliberate, and soul search. It can last up to two or three hours on a nice snowy day, or on a Sunday when there is nothing to do, or on a Tuesday night when nothing is on TV. In the old way, to sit and make prayer is introspection, and introspection is the circle of self-examination.

Find a quiet place where you will not be disturbed. Place your medicine blanket where you can sit. Put a white candle in a candleholder and set it down in a place where it won't start a fire. Say a prayer while you light your candle, thinking of Great Spirit, Grandmother/Grandfather. While sitting on your medicine blanket, perform the Ceremony of the Sacred Herbs, smudging yourself properly, and prepare to answer the following questions in your journal:

1. What is your spirit time? What time of day or day of the week do you perform spiritual activities?

2. On what do you base your physical appearance?
Example: Does someone tell you how to look, how to dress, how to walk, what to eat, how to exercise? Or do you do that?

3. What are your inner needs? Things? Beliefs? Ways of action that make you you?

Example: Money, homes, cars, religion, business, career, titles, people.

4. What is your life to be used and known for?
Example: You are a humanitarian, you are a murderer, you are a good family person, you are hateful.

Answer the questions to yourself, and record them in your journal, so that you have a clear understanding of yourself.

Now hold the blue cloth in your hands and know you are going to tie this cloth onto the stick. Hold the stick and the cloth together and ask yourself the following questions:

1. What do you hate/love?
2. Who are you?
3. Where do you want to be? Where do you want to work, live, visit?
4. How do you see your physical self?

Example: I don't like my hair color, I don't like my size, I don't like my eye color, I like my voice, I don't like my physical.

5. How is your health?
6. With whom are your relationships?
7. What is self-respect for you?

Record these questions and answer them in your journal. If you can't answer all eleven questions, seek counsel from spirit, from elders, guides, family members, teachers, counselors, or doctors. When you have finished asking yourself the questions and writing the answers in your journal, remember that this is your self-analysis, your self-feelings, and you can do this any time you want to, to get in touch with the inner side of yourself.

When you are finished put away your herb bowl and herbs, blow out the candle, put away your journal and pen. Tie the blue cloth onto the stick and place it at your medicine wheel by sticking it in the ground at the West gate. You can also place it on your altar or in a special place in your home where you will see it and remember that you have done your Ceremony of Introspection. Your feelings after the ceremony will be calm. You will be organized and in charge, with your goals understood, and with a good understanding of yourself and your needs.

Ceremony of Intention

TOOLS: *A blue candle (representing your truth and the Proof of completion); a candleholder; a pen and your journal; cornmeal; your medicine blanket; smudge bowl, fan, matches, and herbs.*

You need to find a place to put your medicine blanket where you won't be disturbed. No phones, people, pets, or noise. Set out your candle and candleholder.

The Ceremony of Intention starts with the Ceremony of Sacred Herbs, so smudge yourself, balance yourself by breathing, and become ready to do the ceremony.

You will need cornmeal—any type will do. You put it down to honor the earth. Placing cornmeal, tobacco, or herbs in a ceremony is done simply out of respect as a give-away to all the spirits and others who might be assisting you in the ceremony. If you are doing your ceremony inside, I suggest you sprinkle the cornmeal on the floor in an area where you can sweep it up easily.

Intention is the way you achieve. As you progress in understanding your physical existence within Bone Medicine, the Ceremony of Intention allows you to ask yourself a question: What does this book and these instructions have to do with me, and what will I be gaining from the time I spend reading this book?

Intention has seven sacred movements:

1. To find your purpose. There is a purpose in everything you do—and you need to find that purpose.

> ***Example:*** *An individual is setting out to go to college. That is the purpose—to set out to go to college.*

2. Examine the idea.

> ***Example:*** *I would like to obtain a special license, or teaching credentials. That is the idea I have in my mind right now, because I would like to expand myself. I love to learn and I need to, in order to be respected by my community.*

3. Set goals.

> ***Example:*** *(1) I will do an Intention Ceremony. (2) I will outline the project. (3) I will obtain the financial information I need. (4)*

I will make a commitment to attend and do my best in school. (5) I will learn and graduate.

4. The direction that you will go. This is setting it up so that you know exactly where you will be going and when.

Example: I am going to take two years of community college, because it is less expensive than the regular state school. Then I am going to attend the last two years at the state school. Then I am going to continue on in an undergraduate program to achieve my master's and doctorate.

5. Project organization. Here you actually sit down and make a list of what you will need and how you will get through the project.

Example: (1) The things that I will need to go to college are clothes, money, transportation, a place to live. (2) The steps to going to college are [1] find the school, [2] know what I am going to study, [3] line up my classes, [4] pay for my classes, [5] attend my classes, [6] study the topic, [7] achieve the knowledge.

6. The end in view. This is being able to sit and vision the end of your process.

Example: My first year I don't know much. My second year it's not as scary, because I've been there before. My third year it's all old hat. I know what I'm doing; I have friends; I have a community; I know where I live; I know the grounds and the town that I am in. My fourth year I see myself finishing. I won't be there anymore. I won't be seeing the same people anymore. I see myself graduating, having a celebration, starting to go out for interviews, and achieving the next project I have in mind.

It is important when you do the "end in view" that you actually sit and see it in your mind. If you can't see something in your mind, then you need more counseling, more instruction, and more guidance to understand what you are doing.

The Ceremony of Intention starts with knowing what you want to do. You want to set the movement of your Ceremony of Intention, so that you are constantly aware of what your goals are.

7. Make a decision. A decision is a final point. It's the point before which you step off and achieve what you're after.

> *Example: All of this is just good thought, but physically I am going to go into a world of all new people, in a new place, and it's going to put me in partial or total debt, or I'm going to have to work very hard to get the money, and I am going to spend all the money I work for in order to know something. I like knowing. I want to know what I know. I'm going to do the best I can. I have to seek out anything that I might not understand and sit with it, intentionally, and make a decision if it is what I want to have happen. I don't want to forget the bad things, like I might fail and have to start over again, or things might go up in price and I'll have to work an extra job to make it happen. I can't forget to think about the things that happen like sickness during classes or an accident that slows me down and gets me behind. Am I able to do this? Yes. It's what I want to do. You make your decision and you go about your project.*

Put the smudge bowl beside your candle. Take the blue candle and say a prayer of intention. Light the candle, set it in its holder, open your journal, take your pen, and list the following questions of intention:

1. What is the project title?
2. What tools do you need to do the project?
3. What is the goal you wish to achieve for the project?
4. Who will be involved in the project?
5. Describe the outcome of the project.
6. What are the actions, people, or things that could keep you from achieving your project goal?
7. When will the project be over?
8. Are you sure you want to do this project?
9. What is the "bad" that can be connected to this project?
10. What is the "good" that will come from this project?

After you have answered all the questions, blow out the candle. As you do this, in your mind's eye see yourself achieving the project that you have set your Ceremony of Intention for. Then put everything away.

Spiritual Colors of the Physical Movements

In my personal vision of Rainbow Medicine, the seven stars came to me as seven colors—red, orange, yellow, green, blue, purple, and burgundy. My lifetime of understanding the colors of those seven stars has brought me to the definition of life as simply seven colors. In other words, everything is a color. I have classified life as a color. The study of Rainbow Medicine has given me an opportunity to connect with the vibrational frequencies of a color, and to understand that everything starts with energy. And energy has color, hue, and complexity. It is vivid, in customs, speech, background, and viewpoint. Color is attitude. It is outward appearances. Life is constant, perpetual color (everything, anything, something—all).

I explain the spiritual colors of the physical existence this way: Energy brings particles—some of the extremely small constituents of matter—to life, and the physical existence comes forth as matter. In other words, spirit (unseen energy) expands into visual matter (our physical existence, our human form). Our two-legged form is a metaphysical experience—highly abstract and subtle—which includes the nature of existence; the origin and general structure of the universe; the origin, nature, methods, and limits of human knowledge; the truth and principles of knowledge and conduct.

Our existence is also supernatural, spiritual, and physical matter. Our human life, our physical existence, is made up of seven parts. I would like us to take a look at the seven parts of the physical existence and classify them with spiritual colors. Then we'll be able to see what we can learn about each part of our existence from the color connected with it (a part of the body, for example). We will examine it in view of the color interpretations here (in the Color definitions in the back of the book).

In my vision, each star taught me its definition by telling me the words that apply to each color. Each star is a color that is a medicine word and a lesson word. Each star is a word, each word is energy.

> ***Example:*** *I have applied purple to the body—the body being defined as skeleton, frame, bones, physical form. In applying purple to the bones, for example, you are looking at the real part of yourself. In the same way, you will learn the lesson of complete by understanding your body.*

Allow the colors to talk to you. When I give you a word such as Real or Complete, which are the words connected to purple, you need to study those words. Always when you see a color connected to words in my teachings, study those words—their antonyms, their synonyms, their dictionary definitions, everything you have ever learned about them, and it will enrich you with a rainbow understanding.

The seven movements of physical existence are:
1. **Body—purple** (skeleton, frame, bones, form).
2. **Energy—orange** (breath, temperature, neuro-processes within the brain, DNA, nerves).
3. **Water—green** (fluids in body).
4. **Flesh—red** (tissues, skins, cells, brain matter, hair).
5 **Blood—blue** (vital principle, life).
6. **Muscular—yellow** (organs, veins, protein, nails, muscular structures).
7. **Spirit—burgundy** (soul, chakras, energy fields, beliefs, thoughts, and mind).

Understanding the spiritual colors of the physical existence turns you into a rainbow person. We are star people—a star that is energy, a physical being that is energy, made by Great Spirit.

Teachings of Acceptance

In our physical existence we are either push or pull energy, which means things are either coming or they are going. It means we are either coming or going. Life is made up of many things—actions, movements, projects. We have, as very small ones when we first get here, the obligation to figure out what comes first. All through life we ask the question, "Which came first, the chicken or the egg?" Well, it's simple—acceptance. That's what comes first.

If we look at life without acceptance, we have no life. We are beaten before we ever get started, and then we strike back for the rest of our lives. Acceptance is the act of healing. It is re-forming, flowing, believing and making sense of the circumstances in our lives.

When we start out in our existence, from the moment we take our very first breath, acceptance is necessary. Our body says breathe, and we do. To understand acceptance, look at it as being willing or receptive to whatever comes your way.

Acceptance is a magical word, for it is a mystery. The only time we really understand what acceptance is, is when we do a ceremony and sit down and put things in order, look at our intentions, and understand why we do what we do. In our existence we are faced with lifetime, generation, correlation, longevity, conditions, flesh and blood, and life span. How can we understand any of that without acceptance—which is "I want to." When we come from spirit to be a physical form, each of us has to accept that it is our life. Take it on yourself for a minute to understand that even though you might feel rejected, abandoned, neglected, and that it wasn't your choice to be here—the minute your existence starts, you were willing; you were receptive of life, and that is acceptance. Your spirit is the energy that brings acceptance to matter. Your spirit embraces your physical form.

Throughout our lives, we think some have it better than others. We often think that we can't do as well as others. All can be treated in Rainbow Medicine by understanding that you have a Choice. Any time that you miss out on the movements of your physical existence, which is life, come to the teachings of acceptance. Remember that when you breathe, you are willing; you are receptive; and that you must understand acceptance. Then go to work setting out your projects and lining out your intentions and introspection. This will open doors to sacred existence.

Aho.

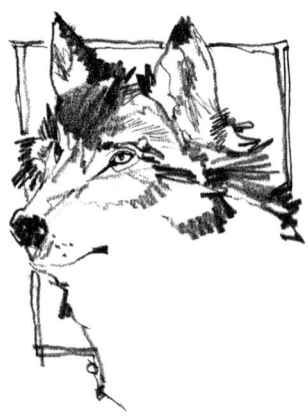

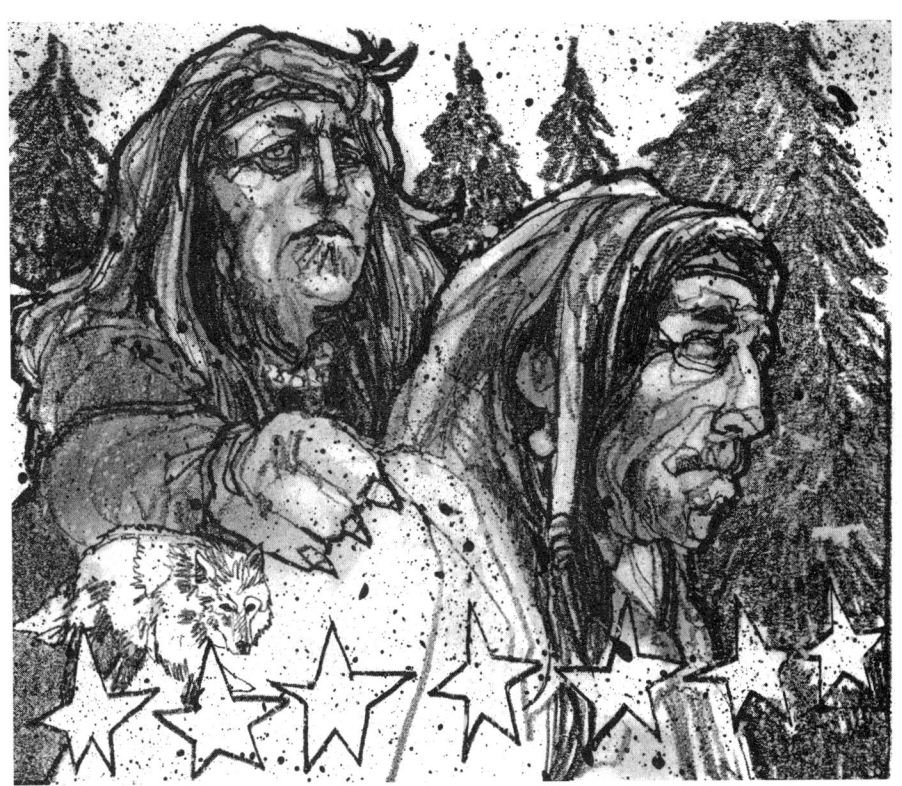

3
OLD WOMAN ROCK—NURTURE

It is dark and quiet. I feel the emptiness sucking my breath away. I feel as if it is turning me wrong side out. I might as well go ahead and roll with it. There is no sense in my thinking that I can teach anything now.

She is gone. Now I am faced with the one thing I fear the most. No elder. No one to turn to. I reach to the side of my waist and pull out my knife. It is sharp. The beauty of its silver blade entices me.

"Grrr." I hear the deep call of a large cat.

The knife is familiar to my hands. "Where is Big Music now? Where is Great Spirit? Make yourself known. Bring your presence here. This is the spirit world. I want to see God and I want to see Great Spirit,

Grandmother/Grandfather, right now. I want to be in the face of the Almighty. All the years of listening to the preachers talk about how comfort comes—that's just words. There is nothing here but darkness and rain. It is Fall—the doorway to death. And I'm sitting in it."

I drop my head and start to weep. Tears run down, dripping on the blade. It might as well be blood.

"Go ahead," says a deep masculine voice in front of me. He springs down from the tree and lands in front of me. A man—tense eyes—a cougar. A four-legged. A two-legged. He stands in all his beauty, golden tan, blond flowing hair and deep, rich brown eyes. He hunkers down.

"I'm not afraid of you," I say.

"No, I can see that," and he starts to circle me. "I can see that you're not afraid of anything, because you're at the crossroads. You'd better listen," he hisses and growls. "You'd better look at me 'cause you're one step into nothingness, and there are only three more to go."

He sits, crossing his legs. His two-legged form is wearing skin pants, and boots made of skin and cougar fur that come up to his knees. I look into his cougar face and his jaws are strong, teeth pearly white. His eyes flicker. He just keeps sitting there with his legs crossed, and his knee keeping time to a beat that I can't hear.

"Do you think it will stop it if you slit your throat, if you drop off into nothingness? Do you think the pain stops? Do you think there is this fairy tale that you can take your life and it's all over?" he asks with a snarl. "Come with me and join the wild. Dare to face the spirit of death. Dare to reach out into the soft nectar of Nurture. Take a chance, make a Choice, make a Change. Oh, I know. Dark Eyes beckons you to dance in the moonlight with him. Dark Eyes, the one with all the answers. Why don't you look him in the face and see if he can answer your grief?"

His tail, in cougar form, swishes back and forth on the ground, making marks in the dirt.

"Dark Eyes doesn't have any answers for me," I say. "I'm not seeking out his dark eyes or looking for anything. I'm just stuck here in this place of emptiness that seems quite familiar to me. I need to go back and tell people that physical form is a wonderful thing, and teach them that life is exciting and joyful even when there is pain and anguish. Just because I am faced with anger and sadness that doesn't mean that life is bad."

"That's it," he hisses. "Go ahead, you're eaten up with it. It's called grief."

I wipe the tears from my eyes. "Of course, it's grief. It's just like the night—it's dark and empty. My mother has died."

"That's right, in physical form your mother has died. But look behind me."

I look up over his shoulder and there is a beautiful blue light—so dark that it is black, blacker than the night itself. A form stands there, and as it moves closer I can see her face—a little scrunched up face with no teeth, that raven black hair and those raven black eyes—old woman that she is. She steps forward.

"Why do you cry, baby girl? Why do you mourn decay and sickness? Don't you understand the heartache? Don't you know what I lived? How they took me from my raven-black-haired mother and locked me in the German Catholic church. Put me away in a boarding school with white people who were not my race. Taught me their language and never mine shall I find. I told you those things when I walked as your mother. That's not who you are here. Look there on the ground beside you."

There was my white tail, lying still in the mud.

"There is no sense in your being this sad. I'm alive. Look at me."

Oh, I remember all the times she used to say that to me. That all I had to do to know the difference between life and death was to look and see if it was looking at me.

"Mom, I'm not ever going to be able to touch you again. I'm not ever going to be able to call you in the middle of the night and tell you my problems, and that is hard. That's really hard for me, because you are my best friend, Mom."

"Ah," she says, with that old sailor growl of hers. "Don't you give me that friend stuff. There is nothing that will nurture you in friendship. Tell her about Nurturing, Golden Heart."

The cougar man looks at me and says, "I am Golden Heart. I am physical existence. I am the spirit keeper of Nurture, and it is mine to tell you that there is only one thing that you can do."

A soft misty rain falls, and I smell the rich aroma of the earth. My mind drifts back to the daylight in the physical realm, the golden trees, the red trees, chrysanthemums of yellow and gold, purple and white, the geese that fly in formation, the golden red-orange sunset and the black silhouettes of trees that kiss the sky. Fall—a favorite time—a quiet time, she used to call it. And the mist shall turn to snow. Death is only snow, she taught me. That's the one thing I remember.

Golden Heart. What a beautiful name. The sternness of his eyes pulls me deeper into his spirit.

I can hear my mother's voice in the wind as it picks up and carries the leaves. "You must learn from Nurture. You must learn to Nurture yourself for it has come my time to stand in spirit form in fullness now."

I hear the flapping of large wings that could only be an eagle flying over me. I watch as it disappears behind me in the canyon. I look into Golden Heart's eyes, and I know that on Earth I will walk alone as a mature adult.

"I have no one to turn to but myself, Golden Heart."

"No, that's not necessarily true. Nurture supplies. It brings forth. When you dry those tears and you stand up, you are nurturing. Follow me," he says, and the cougar turns and runs.

I dash after him with the full force of all the wolf energy I have. We run through the woods. We run across the land, Earth Mother. We run into the sunrise, and into a camp, into a place where an outside fire pit is burning. A wonderful old shack stands in front of me. It is made of wood—logs, pieces of limbs of different trees, all kinds of interesting tin and glass, and boards that are nailed together in artistic ways.

"There. Knock there, and you'll find the Nurture."

I watch him run away behind the rocks and up into the hillside. I step up onto the porch. It is richly decorated with ivies, flowers, and bushes. Flowers are everywhere—pots with geraniums, pots with petunias, pansies, marigolds, chrysanthemums. It is so beautiful with all those colors. English ivy is growing on the side of the house, mixed with honeysuckle and morning glories and every kind of climbing flower that I can imagine.

I knock on the door and it opens. Inside is a quaint, softly warmed little house. Birds are sitting around on different pieces of wood, singing songs. Beautiful rugs made from pieces of cloth and skins are lying about. There are horns, sticks, and dried flower bundles all over the walls, and ceremonial masks made from Earth objects.

"Who's in my house?" a voice calls out.

I look into the kitchen, but there is no one there. The old hand pump at the sink where you can draw up water is vacant. There is no one there. The bed area is the living area. There is no one but me in this square room.

"Hey, you," the soft voice calls out. "Make yourself at home, I'll make some tea."

I look up and there is a banister above me leading to a little loft area to the side, over the living area. A very small area. A very tiny, little house.

"Uh, excuse me," I say. "Are you up there?"

There is no answer. I turn around and there is a huge black dog, wagging his tail. Huge. Very, very huge. He comes up to my waist. Big dog.

"Well, hi, there." I go to pet the dog and he backs up and leaves the room.

I think, well, maybe she's outside. As I step through the front door, I run into a small woman cloaked in a blanket. Her hair is pulled back in a long braid that hangs down her back. It is a mixture of reds, browns, blacks, and whites. She pulls her blanket up around her face, which is aged with wisdom and holds a curious look. Her blanket is shades of red and black stripes, which hang carefully in pleats all around her. She is totally cloaked in the blanket.

"Good to see you, come in—your mother said you'd be here—have a seat," she says in one breath. She starts working the hand pump and drawing up water, fills a teapot and sets it on the wide open stove. Then she pokes a few sticks in the stove. She turns around, waddles over to the rocker, and sits. She kicks off her mukluk boots and wriggles her comfortable woolly socks that are full of holes. Her blanket gives way to an old, full-flowing, denim skirt. I cannot tell what she has on in her shirt area, but I can see a silver necklace.

"Whatcha lookin' at, darlin'? You come for tea, but I think there is more in your heart. You've come for purpose—you want to understand why. You're pretty old for purpose. You should have learned that as a child. You spent a lot of time avoiding your mother dying, and now it's come time and only purpose can tell you that.

"I'll tell you this, my name's Old Woman Rock. I'm going to hand you one object and I'm going to send you off to find your way and purpose. But before you go, I want to tell you a story."

She takes out a small pipe, pokes some herbs in it, lights it up, and smokes. "Why don't you pour us a couple of teas," she asks, pointing

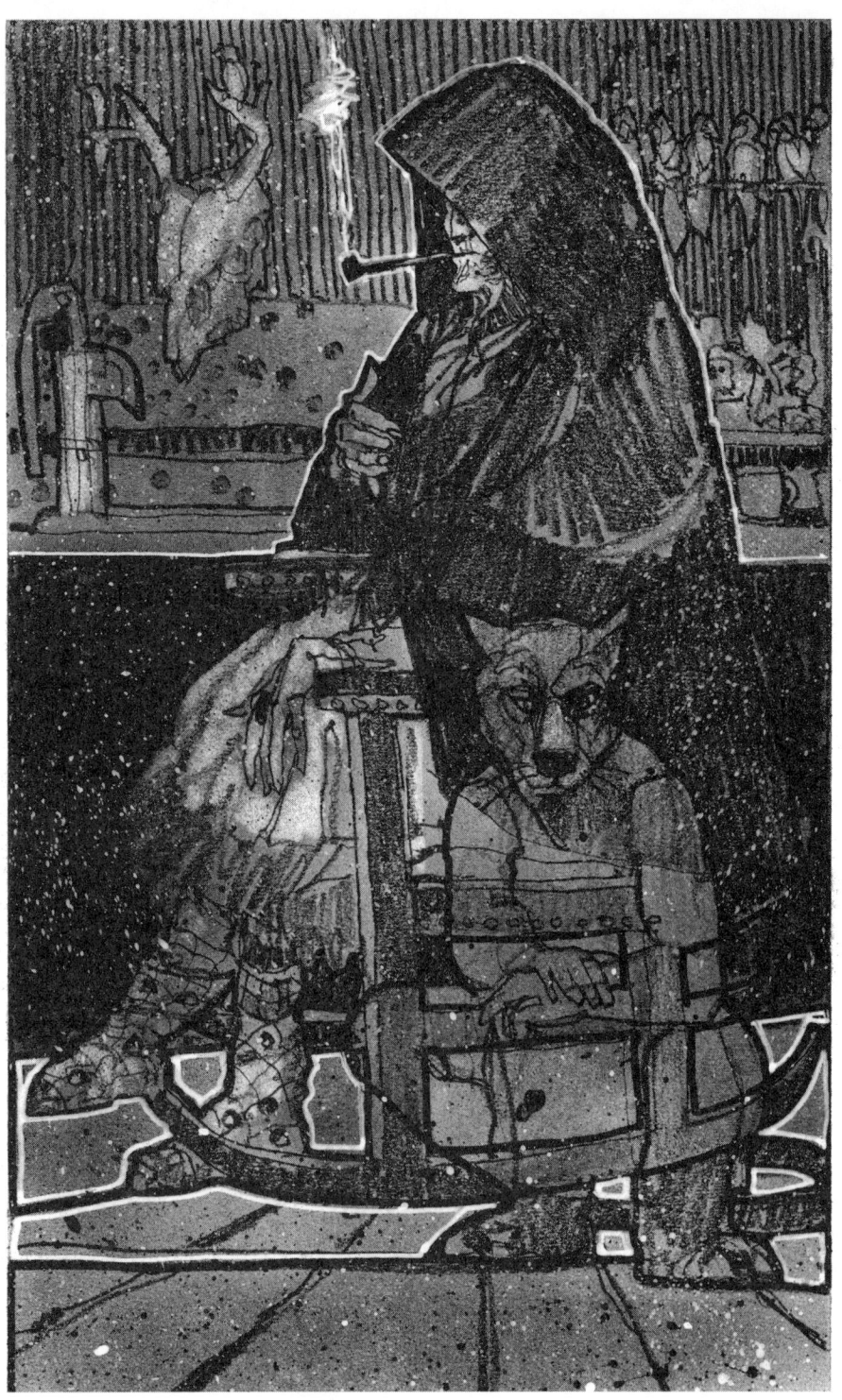

her bony finger at the teapot on the fire. I fix the tea as she speaks.

"Dragon. That's the energy of purpose. The one with the big black eyes, with the red centers and the yellow lines. Dragons. Yeah, ugly old things with filthy breath and long, curved toe nails. Talons, a lot of people like to call them."

She puffs on her pipe and blows the smoke in the air. "Now I don't go out looking for the Dragon of Purpose anymore, 'cause I'm way too wise to have to deal with that old character. When he flaps his wings, he can suck your breath away—he's been known to do that. That will just be fear, you know? Yep. You understanding me? You listening to me? It will just be fear. He's got no power at all.

"The Dragon, the Keeper of Purpose—you want to remember that purpose is a lesson," she says all in one breath, gulping air, and starting up again. "Now he hangs out with a desperate crew. He's got more than one character that hangs out with him, there in his cave. He'll try to convince you that the feeling you're going with is the right one. But his purpose for you is a lie. He wants your life to be a lie. If you live a lie, then you will have no purpose. Better to figure out the difference between fantasy and reality before you encounter purpose, that's what I always say. You will face Choice, and there you will feel the heart of the dragon. You will know if lie is your purpose or if truth is your purpose." She wipes her hand under her nose, takes a big sniff and goes, "Ah. Yep. There's nothing better than some peach tea and a small pipe, and a little bit of talk about purpose to straighten up the fears and the anguish that go along with grief, you know?" she says in an old, crinkly, wrinkly voice.

"Now he oversees the Circle of Darkness and in there is hate and anger and rampage. There is passion and emptiness and ugliness. He specializes, the Dragon, that dark-eyed character, in getting you to understand those are all lessons," and she chuckles with her head back, giving me her old toothless grin.

"How long have you known my mom?" I ask her.

"Well, I've known old Helen for a long time. Yep. Old Crazy Helen, that's what they called her down there on the Earth. The Crazy One is what we call her up here. Crazy Lady. Crazy Woman. We know her. She spins the tales and challenges each one of us. Never a greater spirit have I ever known. Have you?" she says, looking at me with her little scrunched-up eyes.

"Now, Golden Heart wanted you to Nurture yourself and the only way I can figure out how to do that is for you to understand purpose, and it will take you right straight to death and beyond and back. Now you know, down there while you're teaching them students, there is no sense in dillydallying around. Send them to see me and I'll talk to them about Choice. Send them to see me and I'll tell them they need to understand that Old Snake Man—he's had a vision now, he's had a vision. And he ain't wrong, you know? He just ain't wrong. I don't see him being wrong."

She looks over at me. "You want to water them plants on the porch for me? Why don't you get that big old tub over there, fill it up with some water, and take one of them there dippers and dip it out for me?"

"No, now wait a minute, Old Woman. I need to talk about this Dragon and where I'm going."

"Phoom!" I hear a smoke-puffing sound and I am in darkness. Clanking and rattling, gritting of death, moaning and groaning. Spinning emptiness fills my mind. Darkness is everywhere I turn. I hear a deep breath pulling the air from my lungs. I feel an emptiness in every pore and cell of my body. All of my wolf hairs are standing up, and all I can do is pray. I am face to face with purpose. Emptiness, anger, hate, and loneliness.

"The Sacred Circle of Darkness. Welcome."

I hear the rattling of the bones calling me back.

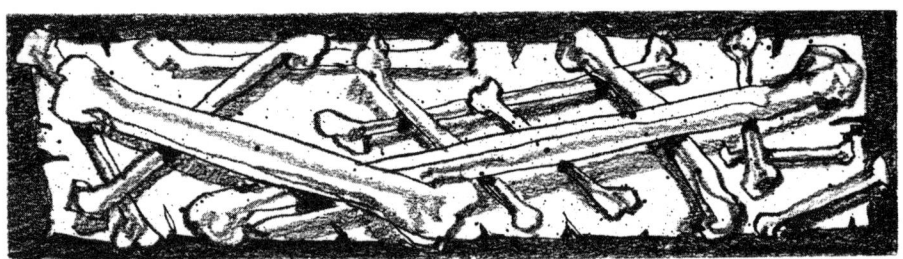

Teachings of Nurture—Cougar Medicine

Often in our lives we think of our purpose as being our emotions, such as anger and fear. Often we feel that purpose is nothing but darkness, emptiness, hate, and loneliness. When we apply the medicine of Nurture to our lives, we put our red to work in the level of our physical existence. Nurture is to nourish, and that is to keep alive. It is to sustain—that is, to support or hold. It is to provide for—that is, to make available. It is to shape—which is outline and organization. It is to educate—which is acquiring, developing—which is effective and strengthening.

These are all terms to apply in your life to bring Nurture forth as a reality. Purpose is strength; it is knowledge; it is effective; it is present and whole. It is life, within life. Everything is at your fingertips when you know your purpose. Purpose is often overlooked. We, as people, don't know our purpose, or don't want to state our reason. We act out of desire and obsession. When we are led by our purpose, we have been taught, we have traditions, we have confidence, because we know what we want. Purpose may be acquired by carrying on your parents' dreams and wishes for you—also by carrying on a family legacy, such as humanitarianism or healing. Your purpose is a knowing, and can come from your visions and dreams. Purpose is your goals, your intention. Purpose is where you draw your strength from. To know the purpose of a matter—or to have a purpose—is the beginning of Nurturing yourself. When we look into purpose, we find it is very spiritual. It is a movement of thoughts that I call pure spirit. When you Nurture and you are a Nurturing person, you are solid in yourself. The teachings of Nurture give us the ability to parent. They give us the ability to guide. It happens in the educational, the developmental part, the providing part of Nurture. When we apply Nurture to our life, we are applying our red medicine from the West section of the Rainbow Medicine Wheel.

You would not be physical without the ability to be Nurtured or to Nurture. Think about the things that Nurture means to you in your life; maybe you'll want to jot them down in your journal.

Example: *Your daily diet, your daily exercise, the beauty you surround yourself with, your scenery, your environment, your education, your teachers, your forms of safety—the people who protect you and watch over you.*

Remember, when you are working with Nurture, that it's not a gun or a knife; it's not a drug; it is others providing education and development, bringing about strength and giving you courage. Nurture is the breath that courage needs in order to live. If you don't have things in your life that keep you alive, that support you and hold onto you when you are weak, you had better go out and get them. You had better reach your hands up towards the sky and reach for Great Spirit, Grandmother/Grandfather, and pray. Find what spirit is.

A lack of Nurture will close down the voice of your purpose. To be supported by a loved one allows us to connect to purpose. When we Nurture self or others, our purpose grows stronger. We achieve our goals when we are Nurtured. So being kind and loving, strong and guiding, helps us all to achieve.

Nurture is your medicine. It helps you to put the silencing moves onto your fear and opens the door to the lesson of purpose. There are many things to learn within the lesson of purpose.

Life Circles—Ceremony of Connecting the Spirit and the Physical

TOOLS: *Cornmeal; pen and journal; Sacred Ceremony of Herbs supplies; gold wire, thread, or string; silver wire, thread, or string; medicine blanket.*

Find a place where you can sit and journal and not be bothered or interrupted. Make a circle with the cornmeal, large enough for you to sit in. Place your medicine blanket on the ground and do your Ceremony of Herbs—smudging yourself by lighting your herbs, placing them in your bowl, and fanning them with your fan or hand to balance your energy. Take out your journal and pen, and journal the following questions:

1. What is spirit to you?
2. Are you whole? If so, what does that mean to you? If you are not whole, what has caused the lack of wholeness? Do you know what wholeness is?
3. What separates your spirit from your physical?
4. Do you understand spirit? List what it is to you.
5. Do you understand physical? List what it is to you.
6. Who can, or has taught you, about spirit and physical? List who and how.
7. Draw a circle and place the following words around the circle.

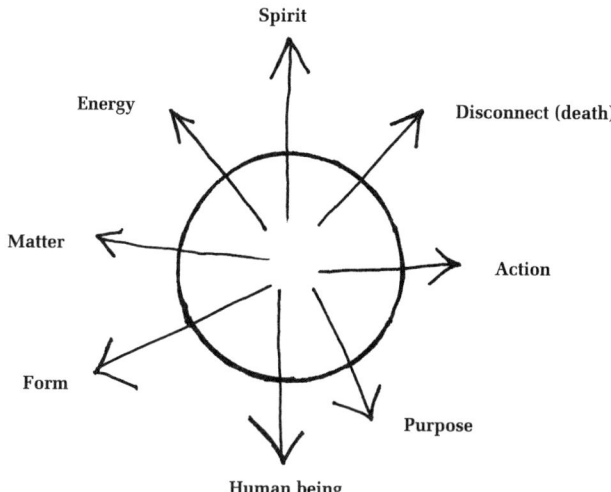

In the second part of this ceremony, take the gold wire or string and make a circle. The gold represents your physical self. Next take the silver wire or string, which represents your spirit self, and run it through the gold circle, connecting them together and making a circle. While you are connecting the circles, visualize your physical and spiritual selves connecting, uniting, and becoming one.

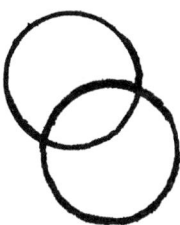

When you have connected your gold circle and your silver circle together, the Ceremony of Connecting Spirit and Physical has taken place in a physical way. Take the physical representation of your wholeness, which is the connecting of your spirit and your physical, and hang it on your wall where you can see it and know it every day.

The third phase—understanding the Ceremony of Connecting the Spirit and the Physical—is understanding that the answers can be found within the seven questions I have asked you. Do you understand each of the words that you wrote around the circle? In your journal write a brief description of each word and how you bring that to life every day.

If you do not understand the seven questions, or you feel you need instructions, I suggest that you connect with someone who can teach you about spiritual and someone who can teach you about physical. Seek out elders and counselors, teachers and ones of wisdom, who can help you understand the depth of these questions.

> **Example:** *You want to be a spiritual person, connected with a spiritual teacher, and you are told to pray and listen to the answer that comes in your thoughts. You are told to follow the good Red Road. This is the answer. This is the spirit. You then give up drinking and wasting time and apply an outline to your life and set goals and work hard to get them. That is physical action.*

When you are finished working in your journal, put your Ceremony of the Sacred Herbs bowl away, pick up your journal and pen, put away your medicine blanket, and leave the cornmeal as an offering to those who have helped. If you are indoors, take up the cornmeal and place it outside as a give-away and honoring to all the spirits and others who have helped you with this ceremony.

Physical Medicine Bundle

To make a medicine bundle, you put together things that are sacred to you, things that help you to focus—objects such as rocks, feathers, sticks, and things that you buy for yourself, such as buttons, hair clips, clothing. Anything that goes into a medicine bundle should help you connect. When you open the bundle, you are making a visual connection by remembering the objects in it.

> **Example:** *You see your prayer ties, remember your prayers, and look into your life to see what the outcome was.*

Think about the objects that are inside the bundle—or just let the energy of the bundle Nurture you. The objects in the bundle will help bring about Nurture. They will give you support, make you feel good about yourself, allow you to have a strong connection with your spiritual voice within.

Keep your medicine bundle under your bed, at your altar, or at a special place in your home where it will not be disrespected. Use it by holding it next to your heart, taking four deep breaths, and asking Great Spirit to tell you what you should do in your daily life.

Building Your Nurture Bundle
Select a piece of cloth or animal skin that makes you feel strong in your physical existence, something that connects you to your body, that says "body" to you. Relate your physical existence to the cloth or the skin.

You can make this bundle as large as you can carry or as small as you wish. The size of a bundle does not affect its power. Remember, dynamite comes in small packages and blessings come in a big way. It is up to you to choose the size of your medicine bundle, the cloth, and the number of objects that go inside.

When you are gathering up the objects for your medicine bundle, pick articles that represent strength, safety, and endurance to you—something that represents keeping you alive, or brings that about—objects that represent the qualities of Nurture. They will educate you or bring about your development; they will provide for you or bring shape to your life; they will give substance, bring about support. These objects are personal to you, therefore I cannot give examples. It is important that you remember to correlate the words with the objects that you put in the bundle.

When you have gathered all the objects you need to put in your bundle, find a quiet place. Lay down your medicine blanket and put the objects and the cloth on the blanket. Do your Ceremony of Herbs, smudging all the objects and yourself. Sit with the objects and start to work. Lay your cloth out straight and pick up each object one by one. In your journal, register what it is for. "I have chosen...[put the name of your object]...to represent...[put what it represents]..." and write down your connection to each object, so that you know its place in your physical existence. Explain each object to yourself—why you chose the cloth that you chose, or the type of skin in which you've wrapped your physical medicine. It is a good idea, when you are choosing the objects, to pick one for each medicine word and each lesson word. This will help you become familiar with your medicines and your lessons.

When you have registered everything in your journal and you feel you understand why you have picked these objects, place them on the cloth. Cover them by pulling the right side of the cloth over them, then the left. Next, pull up the cloth that is left over at the bottom to cover the two folds that you have already made, and roll up the bundle into the remaining cloth at the top.

Once you have rolled up your bundle, you can tie it off with a string. I recommend a colored string that goes along with the physical bundle,

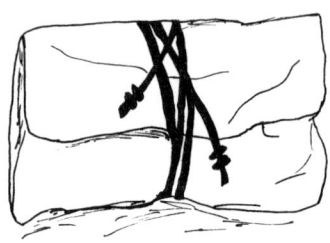

which is blue. You can also tie it with a white string or a black string, white representing spiritual, black representing wholeness.

Your physical medicine bundle is now ready for you to pray with, to place under your pillow and draw strength in dream-time, to put under your bed and listen with your heart when you're resting, to lay on your altar and sit with.

It's a good idea—when you're feeling blue, sad, in grief, anxious, angry, about to give up, suicidal—to get out your medicine bundle, open it, and listen to the thoughts you have about the objects within.

When you are not using your medicine bundle, place it in its sacred place in your home.

Aho.

Process of the Lesson of Purpose—
Teachings of the Dragon

Purpose is the lesson that challenges us in our physicality, in the color red. It is a red lesson from the West section of the Rainbow Medicine Wheel, within the teachings of physical existence. The dragon is the animal totem for purpose. When the lesson showed itself to me in my original vision, the dragon was overseeing purpose because of its steadfast devotion. Dragons have always been known to be loyal. They are a strong symbol for the principle of devotion and for principles themselves.

The lesson of purpose is a seven step process:

1. Spirit. Spirit is the image of Great Spirit (God). Spirit is an animating principle of life. Animating is vital, it is essence, which is substance. Spirit, in other words, is the drawing pool; it is the substance that allows us to achieve personality and character, good and bad deeds, fair and unfair doings, loving and hateful actions, quality, values, principles, rights, and wrongs. If we as human existences draw from spirit, we have our good, bad, fair, unfair, loving, and hateful to choose from—as actions to bring about our qualities, values, and principles. These constitute our rights and wrongs. In other words, spirit can be good or bad, and you can operate in such a way that your physical existence brings harm or does good to others.

2. Vision. Vision is sensing the power of what will come. It is having a dream or a knowing. Our vision is a guide that helps us have goals, points, intentions, by connecting with the knowledge of our vision. Each object in a vision is a guide with an interpretation that helps us make choices.

3. Principle. A principle is the highest in the rank of important values. It is the main value of life (topic, project, action—these are our goals, needs, dreams, and wants). For principle is foremost (the way, path, or belief—these are our medicines, lessons, dreams, and traditions).

4. Cause. Acts that produce a result. Good, significant, reason. Having sound judgment and drawing from the principles that radiate your vision bring you into a total knowing that makes cause an outcome. When you do something, you act upon your qualities or values, along with your principles. The outcome of these thoughts is cause. Motive. Natural flow. When we make right choices that bring happiness to our life, and a good life for those around us, we can see strong natural flow. We should be influenced by family traditions, government stipulations, and our religious atmosphere, assuming that the people involved in these positions are good, loving people and set the highest example. To achieve the purpose of your life, you need to make your own decisions, based on your connection to Great Spirit. Try never to be influenced by others.

5. Devotion. Devotion is an eagerness to be dedicated. It is worship and prayer. Devotion brings about religion, spirituality. You can also commit to being non-committal.

6. **Steadfastness.** Firm, faithful, unwavering, stable, strong. Steadfastness is the ability to be taught and to carry forth the teaching as an action. It is repeating actions from history, which brings about faith. Faith is a cycle of successful movements that bring about a project. Within steadfastness we are unwavering; we never give up; we never stop. We decide on our stable, strong commitment to right or wrong, good or bad, and we use our steadfastness to achieve the outcome of good or bad deeds, loving or hateful deeds, fair or unfair actions, and we represent our spirit in that way.

7. **Reason.** It is results, belief, actions, facts, judgments, good sense, and sanity. In essence we, as two-leggeds, draw our reasoning from what we are taught. Our traditions become our beliefs and they become our causes. Our environment brings about our actions. Our history is our facts. Our ability to look at the things around us is our judgments and the way we judge. Our spirit speaks within our mind, within our brain, and allows us to understand good and bad, giving us good sense. When we follow our good sense, this brings about our reason for action, sane or insane. Reason gives us the outcome of an experience. It is up to us, as physical beings, to learn the lesson of purpose. Often our lives are affected because we have no principles, we are not steadfast, we have no devotion. We don't even realize we are spirit. It is very clear, when we learn the lesson of purpose, that we have connected with tradition, with eldership, and with circles of principles that have existed for many generations.

The lesson of purpose does not mean blood. It does not mean that you have to follow any particular elder or tradition. It simply states that you need to have teachings that bring about good, sound judgments. When you draw upon your teachings, it is necessary to understand spirit, to reflect upon the fact that spirit is the image of God, Creator, Great Spirit, and that we are made as two-leggeds in that image. When we finalize the lesson of purpose in our life, our reason will be a reflection of Great Spirit. We are walking a good life, a life on the good Red Road. We bring honor and respect to ourselves and to Great Spirit!

Aho.

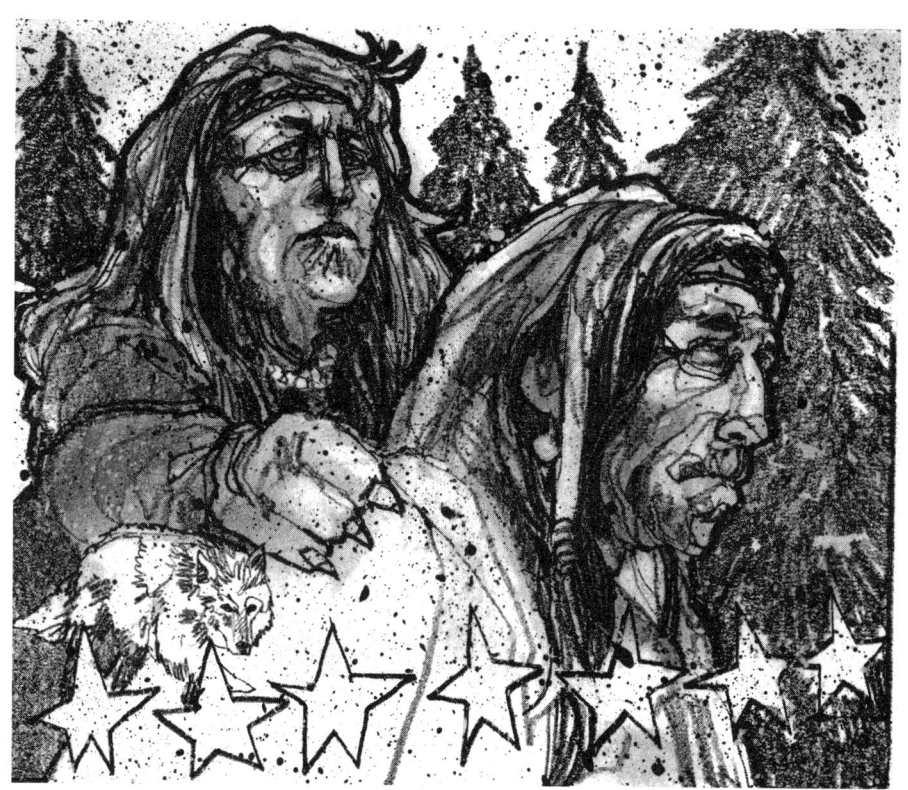

4
THE TURN IN THE ROAD—CHOICE

I sit quietly in the Fall night. What was it that Old Woman Rock wanted me to have? What was the rock that she was going to give me? It's funny, in spirit, how things can flee, and you can never really remember them with your human mind. Looking out over the medicine wheel, candles twinkling in the night, I can see each colored stone. It is very clear; I am in the physical.

But stepping into spirit and making sense of the story that goes on before me is what is hard. There isn't anything in life that is easy—not that I have been able to find. All the grand moments of life and compassion end with sickness and death. Childhood friendships are erased with arguments over a simple marble.

"That's right," a familiar old voice says. I turn quickly and there she is, wrapped in her blanket, standing in the West part of the wheel by the orange stone. She points her finger at the stone and says, "Choice. What was the stone I gave you? It's right here. It's Choice."

There's an enormous flapping of wings over my head and I feel a large dark being descending upon us. Everything is engulfed in its black spirit. Before me, I see an opening in the blackness, and I move into it. I am standing in a cave. A fire is flickering way inside.

"Be careful!" says Old Woman Rock. "To learn Choice and to understand its lesson, which is obedience, you must know what careful is. Careful is the balance within Choice. It is the second movement of Choice—Choice—Choice—" her words echo off the wall of the cave. "You now enter into the mouth of the Dragon. You are going within the depth of purpose. You must understand that—that—that. Wolf—Wolf—Wolf. You'll know me in Ceremony—mony—mony. After me comes Snake Man—Man—Man." Her voice echoes.

"Where am I going, Old Woman—Woman—Woman?"

"Inside purpose, Wolf—Wolf—Wolf."

I walk deeper into the cave and the walls are alive. They twinkle and sparkle with deep shades of purple. It is beautiful. All the shades of purple—light ones and dark ones—glitter from the light that is ahead of me. It is amethyst. All the walls are amethyst. But I'm inside a dragon, I think.

"That's right, you are."

In front of me hangs a bat, staring me right in the face with its tiny beady eyes, and two little fangs at the top of its mouth and two little fangs at the bottom.

It is hanging upside down. It is silver—almost white. It shimmers. Its wings are folded across its chest and it is swaying in the air.

"Hi! Watcha doin' here? I just hang around, that's what I do here. Hi! My name is E.G."

"E.G.?"

"Yeah. Yeah. E.G., that's my name. E.G. Bat."

"You're E.G. Bat Medicine?" I ask.

"No, no, no. I'm E.G. Bat," and with that he flips himself down on his feet and looks up at me. "I'm Obedience. E.G. Obedience. E.G. Bat Obedience, to be perfectly, perfectly clear. That's me. E.G. Bat

Obedience." He opened out his wings and stretches them. "Well, are you ready for Choice?"

"Wait a minute. I want to know what E.G. stands for."

"Oh, that's easy. It's Extra Good. Extra Good. Extra Good Obedience," and he laughs, a small, tinkling sound. "Listen. Listen to me. See, you have to listen to me, because I'm obedience."

"Hey, what's that light up ahead, E.G.?"

"Oh, that's your Choice. You've got to get there. And then, once you're there, guess what happens? The Ceremony of Life!"

I hear a rattling faintly in the distance.

"Yep, yep. That's right. You want to listen for that rattling of the bones because our physicality—this right here," and he claps his wings together, "it is ours to learn opportunity, adventure, everything that life is. You see it isn't just the two-legged who are on this quest, it's all of us, and we have been placed here mmph, mmph, mmph..."

All of a sudden I can't hear him anymore. It's as if somebody put a hand over his mouth and he's continuing to mumble... "Mmph, mmph, mmphmmph. Mmmph, mmphmm, mmph," in deep, loud, short tones.

"Hey, E.G., what are you trying to say to me?" I ask.

He becomes very quiet and just reaches out towards the light. He glances at me with a foreboding, distant look in his eyes, like there is something he wants me to know. He draws in a breath and his little chest pokes out, and he says, "Obedience will tell you the truth. You must make the Choice. You must know the Choice."

With that, there is a tinkling sound and many, many orange stars, and he disappears within them.

"Hello—is anyone there? Where did you go?" I ask.

"I'm here." I hear a new voice say.

"Who's that?" I ask.

"Oh, just me. Just the one you seek. Just the keeper of that," a soft, deep voice says.

I can see the light ahead of me. It is clear. I take a deep breath and it smells like meat, blood—hamburger, roast beef, chicken—like meat, fresh and raw.

"Thump, thump. Lub dub. Thump, thump. Lub dub." The sounds are deep and pulsating.

"I guess I go forward, right? Grandmother! Old Woman Rock! Anybody! Is there anybody there?—there?—there?"

"Yeah, I am. Come here. This is the way. Don't you know?"

"Don't I know what?"

"This is the way."

"Okay, I'll start coming towards your voice."

The voice drifts to the back of me. "Really? You'll come towards my voice?"

I turn around, and say, "Yes, I'll come to you."

The voice drifts to my right side. "Really? You'll come to me?"

I turn to my right. "I'll come that away," I say.

"Really?" and the voice drifts to my back.

I turn. "I'll follow you, wherever it is you're going!"

"Really?—really?—really?"

"Well, make up your mind which way you're going," I shout.

"That way."

I head forward, and the voice says, "No. I'm here," and it is behind me again.

I spin around quickly and say, "Okay, I'll play the game and come that way."

"It's not a game, but it's very good that you'll come to me."

"Great." I look down. "I guess I'll go down, then."

I hear the voice from above me now. "Be careful. Down is not the right way."

"Am I ever going to get to you? I need to see you to know where I'm going or I'll just stay here!"

There is no sound—nothing but quietness. It feels soft and squishy underneath me. The cave isn't a small cave, by any means, and it is cold.

"Hey, E.G., are you there?"

I feel a soft, warm vibration beside my heart. I just know. I know I have to get to that light, and I start to walk.

"That's right, go this way." The voice is in the center in front of me.

I walk and I walk, and soon I come to a fire. It is an unusual looking fire—a large rock-shaped object of reds, and yellows, and hot, hot orange—and it is glowing bright in front of me. I can feel air pulsing in and out.

Beside the rock-shaped object a figure stands—dark and tall, cloaked in mystery.

"Welcome," it says. "You are inside your purpose. Do you know your purpose?"

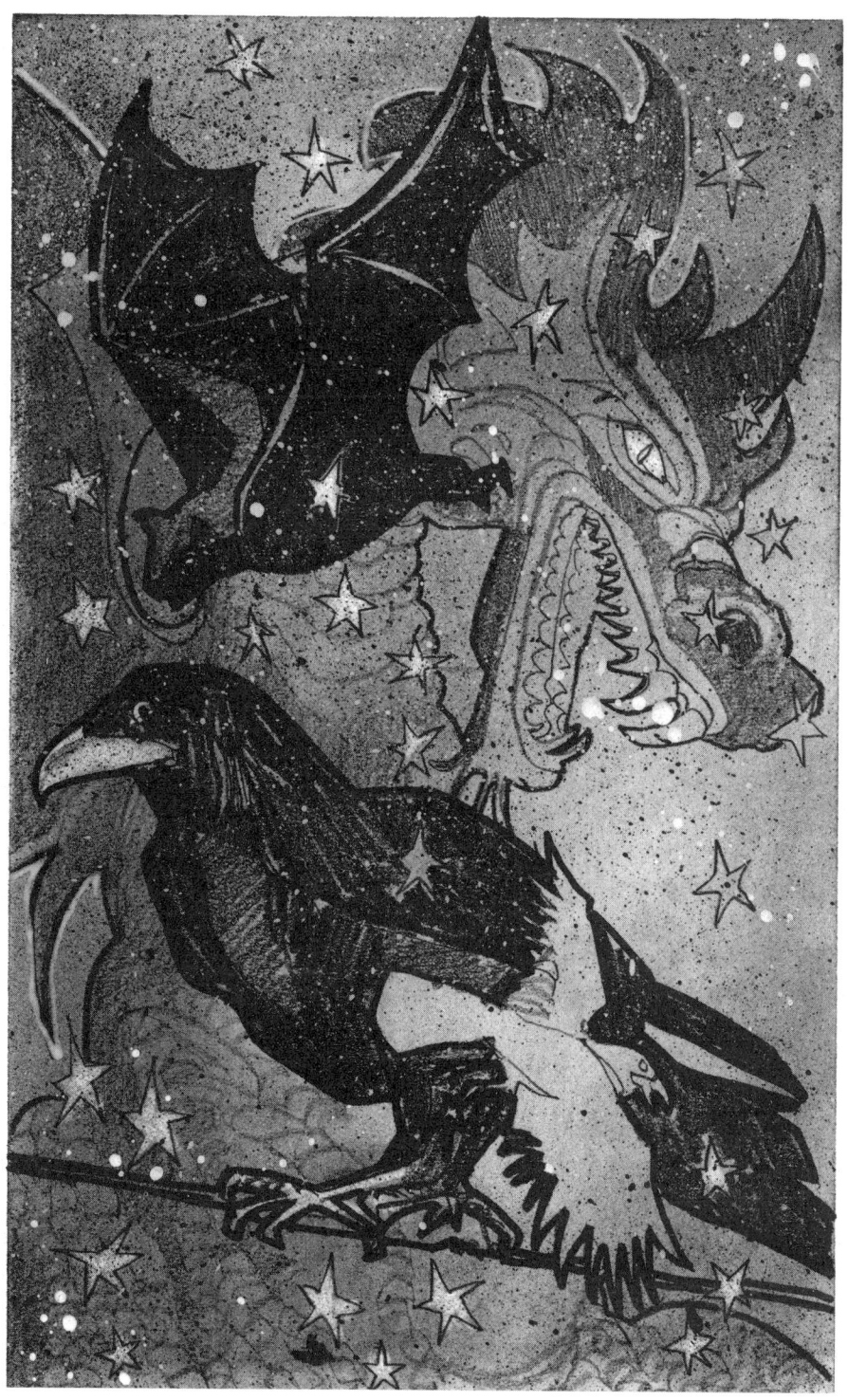

Soft music is all around, beautiful sounds. I can hear the clicking and rattling of bones. There is vastness—I look up and there are stars.

I'm standing on a hillside, with tall ponderosa pines around me, looking out over everywhere—land is all the way around me. The campfire is glowing, and there stands the dark silhouette. I cannot see his features. I can tell only that he is male. I can tell only that he is present.

"Nothing more do you need to know from me, for I am the Blue-Eyed Raven. Do you know your purpose?"

Never have I heard such a soft, beautiful voice.

"Purpose is hard, Raven. It's hard for me to understand."

He points towards the North. As he swings his arm around, colored stars fall from his winglike sleeve. The stars scatter to the ground and bounce. "It has been said that the Raven is the one who brought mankind to Earth. What is your purpose?"

"Well, somebody has to take care of those stars. They're just rolling down the hillside, Raven."

Man, what an awesome sight! The stars bounce—some zip, some shoot away, some spin and soar, run and jump, and some move along slowly. They each have their own unique individual way. They seem to just come down from the North and drip out his sleeve. They hit his hand and fall on the ground.

"Those are beings," he says in his soft voice. "They have come here to Earth Mother. Here, right underneath our feet."

I look around and it is familiar. Just ahead of me and down a ways is the medicine wheel.

"I'm on the Earth, and you're here with me?"

"Oh, no. You're deeper than that. Remember, you made a Choice. You once came here the same as your students do. You followed your vision and it's taken you inside of purpose, and now you're here with me. I am the Keeper, also, of the West. It is my job to see to it that creation understands its existence. I guess you could say the Raven's job is to point out the story, to show the way, to keep you comfortable and as safe as I can."

He takes flight, singing out his strong caw sound, and circles above me.

"Hey, wait. I'm not done asking questions."

He flies away down the canyon, singing his song as only a Raven can.

"Great! Here I am again. I have journals that speak of jealousy, sickness, sadness, and evil things that have happened to my students. I have students who are addicted, students who use liquor and drugs and smoke tobacco, students who are scared, students who are nervous, students who have plenty of money, and students who have a good life—students with success and students looking for success."

"Yep. Yep. That's a shaman's job." There, hanging in the tree, is E.G.

"Do you always hang upside down?"

"Yep. And I hang upside down extra good, too. That's how I get my name—E.G. How do you like obedience? Isn't it fun, how it just kind of drops in on you? Isn't it fun to understand that your whole purpose is to live for other people and deal with their problems?"

"Oh, yeah, it's great," I snicker.

"Having a little trouble with obedience, Wolf?"

"I've never met a person who didn't have trouble with obedience. I thought that being spiritual would make a difference, but obedience teaches me that—"

"I don't think obedience has taught you anything yet. I can tell you where to look for it, though," he says. "Your Proof. Don't be afraid of obedience, Wolf. When you have it, it is Proof."

"I came to the spirit world looking for that very thing, E.G., Proof."

I feel myself shaking inside, and a coldness comes from my back. My jaws get tight, and I sense extreme heat in my face.

This is confusing, I think. "I don't like this feeling, E.G. It happens every time I try to be obedient."

E.G. swings back and forth and says, "No."

I stand very still and the shaking gets stronger. The coldness is all around me now.

"You must choose," E.G. says. "Remember Choice, and I would advise you to do it quickly."

I watch him close his wings around his head to hide his face.

"Oh, no," he mumbles. "You're going to blame me again! Evil," he says in a small voice. "Think about it, Wolf. Everything is backwards here. Spell it."

"Great. I flunked spelling."

"Spell it."

"E—V—I—L. There!"

"No, backwards!"

"You want me to spell 'backwards?'"

He takes his face out from under his wings and says, "Evil—say it backwards."

"Hmm," I say. "L—I—V—E."

Immediately I'm normal. I feel great.

E.G. flies around me quickly—just sparks past me. He lands in the other tree and says, "A wolf and a bat and a raven. We're the three most evilest things that exist. They talk about us like we're just pure Hell itself. Legend says the wolf is a beast that lurks in the night and rips out the throat of the innocent. Legend says the bat is the vampire that transforms from physical to animal form. Raven is said to be the grandest of all tricksters, who lures you into insanity. Great crew, huh?" He laughs.

"Gee. I—wow—I don't think I chose this group and I don't remember being those things. I remember living my whole life trying to keep the lessons of goodness and follow the circle of right. But I guess there have been times that you could say I do rip throats out."

"How come?" E.G. asks in a faint little voice, his head tilted to one side. "How come they speak of us like they do?"

"Well, it is easy to call something you are afraid of evil," I say. "The bat is mystery, and the wolf is power, and those things scare the two-leggeds. The raven is black and has often seemed evil to humans. So lots say we are the symbol of evil, when we are just a wolf, a bat, and a raven."

"Absolutely," E.G. says, with a squeaky tone in his voice. "Don't you think we choose sickness? Don't you think we choose evil? Don't you think we choose what we do?"

"Well, well, that's a hard one," I say, stuttering. "I—I don't, you know, think I ever chose anything that happened to me."

"Oh, poor, poor, little girl. I guess you was a rare one and everything just happened to you, right? Do you know the wolf's best friend?"

"Hmmm. Can't say that I do. Can't say that I ever believed in friendship. Can't say I'd ever want a friend, because they just let you down. Can't say that I would even participate in that word. I've been around enough to know that friends aren't worth the salt it would take to make a dinner taste right," I say.

"Ah, don't be so hard, Wolf," E.G. said. "Friends are great. They're opportunity, just like life. You're going to see that by the time you get to Grand, when you meet up with Grandfather Ram—he's going to be so proud of you, because physical existence is an opportunity, it's an adventure. It's the ability to prove that you are the image of Spirit. Spirit has no fear of friends. It takes them for how they are and it..."

"Hey, hey, hey. Wait," I said. "I'm not taking anything from anybody. I know what it is. There are no friends. In my physical existence, my parents were supposed to be the greatest friends you could have. Parent is supposed to be a word of safety and guidance. For someone to be a guide, they have to be safe, because otherwise you'll get..."

"What?" E.G. asks with a questioning look. "Hurt? You might learn something? Hurt is just a lesson. All these things in life—people make them so, so big."

"Hey, E.G. I work with doctors and therapists all the time. People have always known abuse and distress to be what they are. Hurt. Pain."

"Oh, yeah, yeah, yeah," he says, in his tiny voice. "Hurt and pain. Hurt and pain. How come people can't see friends and family, pain and hurt, as green? How come they don't know it like it really is? Snake Man can tell you. He can tell you what green is. He's had a vision, Wolf. He knows. He knows, because he watches over green, blue, and purple. He knows his medicines in the West. He knows what physical existence is about, and you're going to go and see him, 'cause you don't have any Choice. You're on your way to Grand."

"Where is it that I signed up for all this? I don't remember. You know, I was minding my business and I caught chicken pox, and then the next thing I know I'm having this vision. Then before I know it, I'm following this vision."

E.G. laughs. "Hurt and pain. . . Let me show you who I really am."

He takes flight, and in front of me are these beautiful orange stars. They scatter among the trees, little points of light on every branch, on every limb.

"Orange Stars is who I am, Wolf. Who are you? Do you remember? Do you know what band you are from, and what clan you are from? Yeah, you're a wolf, but what color?"

I take a deep breath, and let it out. "I don't know. I don't know. I guess I'm white, 'cause I deal with everything."

There is no answer.

"I guess I'm just pure white, like a white wolf ought to be. I don't know—that's a good question, what color I am."

"Hey, do you know your totem? Do you know who your inside animal is? It's not a wolf. You've got a guardian who watches over you. You got any idea who that is?"

"Well, I don't have a guardian," I said. "I don't need one. It's like friends. The whole time I've been on Earth, everything has always hurt—every friend has always gone their own way, everything has always been a part of..."

"Abandonment, maybe?" a soft, clear voice says from behind me. I look and there is the dark figure. "Maybe it's all about abandonment. Maybe you can't see past your humanness into your spirit clear enough. You need a strong, clear spirit voice to teach," I hear the dark figure say.

"Hey, are you Raven?" I ask. "It's all just talk. I love to talk," I chuckle. "Wolves love to run along and share their knowledge, that's one of their best personality traits, and I'm just a natural gabber. As a human, I like to talk."

"Yeah, I know that about you, and what you say makes good sense, because no one should lean on words. People should know spirits. You made a Choice, Wolf, and the only thing I can say is, you're not alone. I think you're reacting from Dark Eyes. I think you're finally going to get that mystery figured out."

A quietness is all around me. The soft night breeze floats from tree to tree.

"Dark Eyes," I think. "That's the only friend I know. He's always been there—to hate, to love, to argue with, to gain strength from—he's always been there."

There is no sound. A sadness comes over me. No matter how hard I try, I feel only emptiness.

"Maybe—maybe Dark Eyes is not even real," I say. "Maybe he's just a figment of human imagination. Yeah, like everybody in the spirit world—what's a figment of imagination, anyhow?" I ask. "Who are you? Are you the Blue-Eyed Raven?"

"I am Choice," the figure says. "I think Dark Eyes is real to you and it is important to answer the question 'Is your spirit real and is real physical?'"

I hear the rattling of the bones calling me back.

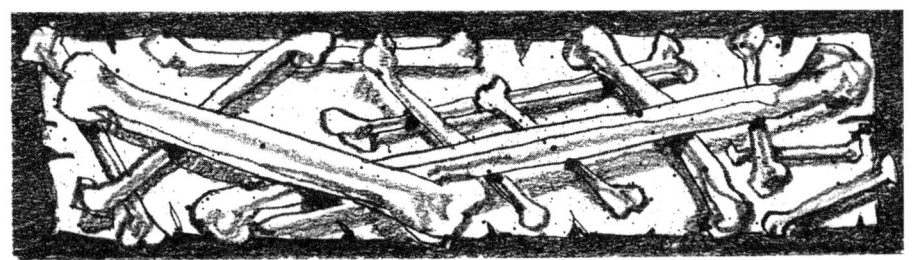

Teachings of Choice—Raven Medicine

When Choice emerges in our physical existence, we have opportunity. Choice is a form of the perpetual circle, which means it is constant Change. You can't have Choice without Change and you can't have Change without Choice. They belong to a sacred movement of four, which is reason and Choice, Change and chance. In that sacred circle, opportunity comes forth. I wish that I could paint a picture clear enough for you to see reason and Choice, Change and chance, but there are no material things that can help you see that.

Reason brings about Choice; Choice brings about Change, and Change gives you chance. You move that along in any direction—Choice brings about reasons; reasons bring about Change and Change is a chance. Chance is the reason that gives Choice to Change. Change is the reason that you have Choice as a chance. These movements in life are all a part of opportunity. Choice is a medicine, and if you apply it to your life, you give yourself a doorway of movement any time you need it.

If you don't like something in life, make a Choice. Choose, which is a Ceremony, and Change happens, and that's a chance—you have an opportunity at that point. That can be seen in lots of things we do in our lives. Life is constant Change, Choice, chance, and reason.

Choice is an act. It is instant, which makes it spontaneous. In other words, Choice never stops; it is perpetual; it is constant. The sacred movement of Choice is:

1. Right. We always hope we make the right choice. We are always moving in a right way for Great Spirit created us, Great Spirit loves us, and Great Spirit always holds us in its hand when we are two-legged.

2. Careful. When we move to careful, we slow down. Careful can be looked at as planning, as goals, as organizing. To be careful is to be connected, to have respect and intention.

3. Discernment. We have the ability to perceive, to judge, to question, to find. It is a gift to know and see things the way they really are.

4. Opportunity—to adapt, to plan and dream, to know you can achieve anything you set out to do, to take upon, to call forth, to summon.

5. Selection. Our will of spirit is our ability to select our path. We each have a free spirit to draw energy from. The will of our spirit is our inner voice, the voice that tells us what to do, how to act in life, and what choices to make. Our spirit gives us a constant, eternal—a forever ability—which is the will of spirit.

6. Power is knowledge, learning, knowing, conceiving, taking on. The more we experience, the more power we have.

7. Worthy. Excellent, Grand, doing right by others, serving and showing worth and know-how. Living our experiences, living the teachings of our teachers.

When we look at the teachings of Choice, it is important to remember that making a right decision, being careful about that decision, and always having an alternative to that decision, give us opportunity. When we make a selection, we use a power that comes from being worthy. Our Choice comes from having a worthy selection.

A Choice is a worthy thought, if it is a good Choice. To walk a good physical life, you need to know you always have Choice. When we have worth—which is knowing, intelligence, creative thinking—we choose with a good foundation. If we have no worth, we walk as broken people. We often hurt others and ourselves.

To empower ourselves with Choice is a true doorway (a golden one). A right Choice is an organized one. You know what you are going to do by experience, and also what you don't want to do.

Choice is discernment—to perceive and judge your Choice. When we, as two-leggeds, apply Choice to our lives, it is an opportunity to adapt to our moment.

In your selection, the power to move or stand still is yours. I feel Choice is worth. It shows you what you are worth by how you act, by how you bring life forth to live. Choice is a spiritual voice that guides our physical form. There is always a Choice.

Aho.

Ceremony of Choice—the Ceremony of the Broken Stick of Forgiveness

TOOLS: *A forked stick, two to three feet long (60–90cm), with a forked end; red cloth, 100% cotton; blue 100% cotton cloth; seven colors of embroidery thread—red, orange, yellow, green, blue, purple, burgundy; one white candle; cornmeal; your journal and pen; smudge bowl and sage for the Ceremony of the Sacred Herbs; your medicine blanket.*

The Ceremony of the Broken Stick of Forgiveness is an opportunity to clear your mind and forgive. When you are making Choices, it is important that you have a clear mind. Don't carry along any extra thoughts—often called extra baggage. The Ceremony of Forgiveness is a time to dismiss. In your physical existence, most illnesses come from being angry, feeling controlled or manipulated by another, feeling that you don't have control of your own life. Often we reach outside of ourselves and give ourselves away to someone else, allowing them to control our thoughts. To forgive is to let go. The biggest part of this ceremony is letting go. To look at the moment and accept the anger, the fear, and your needs. When you clear your mind, half the battle is over. You must remember that, to forgive others, you must forgive yourself first.

This ceremony should be done outside in the brightness of the day. The best time to perform it is around noon. It is important to let go of anger and brooding emotions, so that your feelings are clear, like a bright blue sky.

1. First, to begin the ceremony, find the stick. Pick a stick that fits your circumstances.

> **Example:** *If you want to forgive someone you're angry with, pick a very gnarly, twisted stick to represent your anger.*

Most of the ceremony of dismissal is to remove one memory and dismiss it. To release the anger, snap off a piece of the stick that you no longer need. Then replace it by drawing in a fresh breath and wrapping the stick with the promises that you make to yourself. Commitments and prayers are represented by the color of thread that you tie onto the stick.

2. Find the place. Look for a beautiful spot in which you can sit and not be disturbed, where it will be quiet and you can do your work. You may need to take a trip or take a vacation. Go to a place like a state park or along the ocean—someplace special to you that is outdoors, to achieve your ceremony.

3. Draw a circle. When you find your sitting place, take your cornmeal and make a circle in which you can place your medicine blanket. You are giving away the cornmeal to the crawlies and winged ones, and to the Earth, out of respect for the work that you are going to be doing. Place your white candle in the candleholder on your blanket and, sitting quietly, light your candle in prayer. Perform your Ceremony of the Sacred Herbs. Take out your journal and list all the things that you wish to put into the stick and break the fork for.

4. Take the forked stick. Start by looking at the path that you have come up, which is at the bottom of the long part of the stick. Move your eyes along the stick and see where you came to a Choice. It is very important to understand that you have control, always. You make the decision about whether you are going to be angry, hurt, or afraid; whether you are going to hold onto it, whether you are going to harbor grudges and feel sorry for yourself, or whether you are going to let go of it, dismiss it, and forgive. The Ceremony of the Broken Stick of Forgiveness is a physical ceremony. It is something that you can hang onto for the rest of your life and remember that you have performed this ceremony.

5. Journal. Now you have your circle drawn, and you are inside it with your journal and your supplies. You have your white candle going, and you are very clear in your mind that the ceremony is a dismissal ceremony.

> ***Examples of dismissal:*** *Memories of an unhappy childhood, memories of divorce, memories of abandonment, memories of decisions that you feel were wrong, memories of lost jobs, wrong decisions you made about those you associated with—these are some examples of things that you can choose to dismiss.*

After you have done your journaling, examine the fork of the stick. Find the side of the fork that represents those pathways. Decide on which side of the forked stick is going to be the "bad" things that happened in your life, things that displease you, or bring you sadness—the things that need to be dismissed. When you have chosen that piece of stick, it is time to write down in your journal that you are going to let go of those thoughts, and you are going to replace them with medicines that you are going to apply to your stick.

> *Example:* You had a bad marriage and you choose to wrap your stick with the blue thread, which represents the truth of the whole situation—how you made bad situations and bad choices, and how it was wrong from the beginning or how it was right and it failed—and you chose to leave. Wrap your stick with the color that strengthens the choices that have been bad for you.

The next example shows how to apply creativity that helps you forgive and forget your bad choices.

> *Example:* You had a bad childhood and you are going to wrap your stick with yellow to represent the creativity in your ability to go on and make better choices in your life—and not to do unto others as was done to you.

6. Wrapping the stick. You can wrap your stick with as many colors as you wish. Each color represents a medicine that treats a bad choice, or a choice that was made that you would like to forget and offer forgiveness to. You can look in the back of the book under the Medicine section and find the different colors that apply to the different medicines you want to incorporate into your life. You may use as many wrappings of each color as there are words within the color.

> *Example:* You might wrap with red, and then leave a space, and wrap around with red again and leave a space, and wrap around with red a third time. The first red represents confidence, the second red represents strength, and the next red represents Nurture.

You can put the wrappings on the stick in different places, or put them together by simply leaving a space in between. It is okay to wrap your stick all in one color, or in white or black. Black would indicate that you are dismissing your bad choices, letting go of the situation, and experiencing the wholeness that is represented by black. White would indicate that you are going to leave it to Great Spirit and let it go. You may wrap the stick all the way down, or you may decide to wrap only

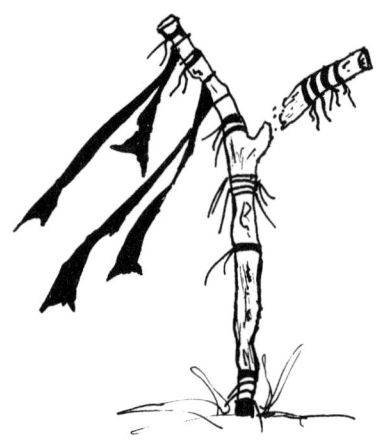

a small spot with the bands of color. Look at the example in the picture shown here to complete your stick.

7. Tying the cloths. When you have finished listing everything that needs to go into your journal, and you feel that your stick is wrapped appropriately, look at the stick and the new medicines that are the path that lies before you.

Take a piece of red cloth and a piece of blue cloth. Cut the cloth an inch wide by twenty-four inches long (1.25 x 60cm). Tie the cloth at the top of your stick—first the red for the Red Road to express your spiritual ability. Next tie the blue for the Blue Road, which represents the physicality of your existence. Tying these two colored cloths on your stick gives you the ability to understand that you can walk the good Red Road and make spiritual decisions that affect your Blue Road, which is your physicality.

When you have finished wrapping the stick, place it on your altar, or inside your Medicine Wheel at the center stone, or hang it on the wall in your home, to remember. Take the unwanted memories—the piece of the stick that has been broken off—and bury it, burn it, or cast it into the water and let it go. At the time you break the fork off the stick, the ceremony of wholeness, forgiveness, and dismissal has begun. I suggest that you remember the broken stick, and think of good things. Connect these good thoughts to the stick, and each time you are tested, remember your good thoughts by viewing the stick.

Begin going forward and fill your life with new dreams, new hopes, and new times. For when you offer a Ceremony of Forgiveness (dismissal) to the Great Spirit, you have altered your path from the old ways and brought about the new ways that Great Spirit, Grandmother/Grandfather wish to give you.

Remember to sit in prayer and to feel the strength of the broken stick. You have dismissed the part that is no longer with you and now you are a clean path of medicines—teachings that come from Nurture, Choice, Ceremony, Change, Proof, Real, Grand, and from other teachings that you may have chosen from the medicine colors in the Rainbow Medicine Wheel.

Aho.

Ceremonial Medicine Pouch of the West

A medicine pouch is something in which you keep symbolic objects. These symbolic objects are connected with your medicine beliefs, your ability to connect a word and a color to an object.

Example: Crystal—*clear, perfect—connected to the word Proof, which means Proof is clear, and it is perfect. It generates energy of that quality.*

Making the Medicine Pouch

A medicine pouch is a little bag, and you can look at the illustration below to see what it looks like. Just cut a piece of cloth, folding over the top and stitching it, so you can draw a string through the opening

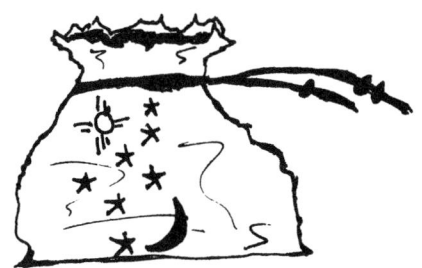

and gather the bag up.

It's easy to make a medicine pouch. You can use the skin of an animal—which needs to be light in color—or you can use blue cloth. You would choose a blue cord for a drawstring. For the neck of the bag, you can use blue, or a silver cord or chain, a light-colored skin, or a white string. The cord for the medicine pouch can be as long as you need it to be for the pouch to hang around your neck and over your heart.

One of the things to remember about a medicine pouch is that it does break; it does come undone, and things do fall out—things move on. We are on a circle in life and things are always moving on. When you lose something from your pouch, pay attention to where you lost it, because that will tell you about an incident that has taken place in your life. You will learn what medicine you need to apply to your life from the color of the object that fell out. You will know this color by how you connected the object to the medicine word when you placed the object in your pouch.

Example: *You are getting a divorce and it is very stressful. You place one stone in your pouch to represent you, and one stone to represent your half-side (your spouse). You wear the pouch for weeks. One day you open the pouch to pray. You go to hold your half-side stone, and it is gone. You then know that the divorce is the right thing for you to do. Your half-side's stone being gone tells you it is over.*

Filling the Medicine Pouch

When you have your medicine pouch, you can put beads on it or things that have to do with the West, raven, black horse, white bear, brown bear, or black bear. Also the symbol of humans, of two-leggeds, bones, and seeds, representing harvest from growth. All colors should be included. Your red objects might be beans to Nurture you. Orange objects might be two of something—two seeds, two rocks, two beans, two peas, or two kernels of corn—to represent the Choice. Your yellow object could be corn kernels, yellow in color, to represent the Ceremony of Life. Your green might be a leaf to represent the Change that takes place in our lives. Your blue object for Proof could be a crystal to represent the clear value, principles, and understanding of life. Your Real object could be a piece of bone that represents purple. Your Grand object might be a star that is white or silver. It represents the Grandness in your physicality and your life after death.

When you have gathered these objects, place them in your pouch, along with a pinch of sage, a pinch of sweet grass, a pinch of tobacco, and a pinch of cornmeal, preferably white. You may place these objects in a small piece of red cloth and wrap them, if you wish, before you put them inside your medicine pouch. I suggest your medicine pouch be no bigger than two inches long by one inch wide (5 x 1.25cm). You can also purchase a medicine pouch, as long as it is either all seven colors or has the seven colors on it, or it can be black or white. The light color is better.

When you have placed all your objects in the pouch, hold your pouch close to your heart and pray for the understanding of your physical existence. Place the pouch around your neck and remember you have your medicine pouch of the West to guide you and help you through your life. You may take your medicine pouch off when taking a bath, but keep it close by. I recommend you never take your pouch off—just wear it until it needs to be replaced. If you should pass away in your physical existence, it's a good idea to have your medicine pouch buried with you. You can give your medicine pouch away, but you must also pass along the stories that go along with the items that are within.

Aho.

Process of the Lesson of Obedience—Bat Medicine

Many times in life we think we are doing what is right, and we call that obedience. Just like E.G. talked about, the bat, the raven, and the wolf are seen as evil. But what is evil? It is Choice. I do not say that Choice is evil—I say that evil is a choice.

If we wish to think of a wolf as evil, the way I look at life, we have limited ourselves to being less powerful than the wolf. We have the ability to outthink the wolf, the raven, or the bat. To be obedient is to know. Like everything in life, we can distort the truth. The act of obedience is to believe in and to follow what we believe in. When people are afraid of something, evil is at hand. The wolf, the bat, and the raven have been chosen to become symbols of evil, when the truth is that people are just scared by them. That is an example of obedience to me—being able to know the truth. It's hard to understand obedience, because it is the act of submitting to authority. Obedience can be seen in your mind as a blue bubble, for obedience is a sphere. That sphere is Truth. You cannot have obedience, nor can you be obedient, unless you know the truth. As a lesson, you must learn to practice obedience in your life, which is to know the truth. To know the truth and follow it is obedience.

It is important to understand that obedience is opposite to negativity, evil, and fear—opposite to anything that brings about our being scared. As two-leggeds, we need to know that being obedient is following the sacred truth. Fear is a natural reaction to protect us in life, but fear does not constitute evil. We could be obedient to evil, but I would suggest being obedient to truth. Obedience is knowing. We make the choice.

If you have seen a bat change into a vampire, if you have seen a wolf change into a werewolf, if you have seen a raven change into a demonic being—in reality, in physical form, where they have left footprints and have a fingerprint, a birth certificate, and a driver's license, and they are a person—then you are truly a fortunate individual, for there is no such thing in reality as something that changes physically into something else. And there is no such thing in reality as evil.

Great Spirit has given us creativity and the ability to talk. As we speak our opinions, we are all writers—we all create. In every race, for some reason, mankind has created something it is afraid of. We must be careful not to live in fantasy, for as writers, we create horror as well as religion. You need to be careful of your instincts, because they will tell you to be afraid. This might save your life in some circumstances possibly—but not, fear of vampires, werewolves, or demons! Maybe we should see the wolf as it is—knowledge, experience, and intensity. And the raven as thought, empowerment, and sacred. And the bat as mystery. When we follow the good Red Road, we don't have to be careful about the dark.

It's time. It's time that we look at our opportunity in the process of the lesson of obedience, to understand the words that make up obedience.

1. Knowledge. The more you know, the more you will see, hear, and understand. This is tricky, because we have to admit that sometimes what we think is physical reality is only in our mind's eye. Therefore, it is pure spirit.

2. Acceptance. To follow or believe in, to give power to something. It is ours, within our own opinion and within our own knowledge, to choose to believe in things that are scary or things that are safe.

3. Adaptability. To change your way into another way. This is where Choice comes in and you can see it very clearly. Often we take on personalities that allow us to fit in with our group. We do what others do in order to belong. It is easy to follow the crowd, to adapt in a safe way.

4. Gentleness. The movement of soft and easy. Sometimes we want to think of evil, and of turbulence and disturbance, as something that strikes fiercely and quickly. It is important to know that gentleness has two sides—one of them the dark side that sways our minds. It is important to bring goodness and kindness to gentleness.

5. Respect. When we choose to be obedient, we show respect to all. Sometimes respect means being quiet, for what someone is doing is not your way, but that person may have his or her own ways and lessons to learn.

6. Passivity. Letting the lessons come, and realizing that the lessons in your life are hard, but understanding them provides a safe space. Sometimes our lessons are horrible. Sometimes they are very, very hard and brutal. Sometimes they are gentle and passive, kind and easy.

7. Faithfulness. Strict, true, promise, and steady understanding. The movement of faithfulness will bring you to a level of impeccability that opens your physical being to Grandness. Life can be hard, due to the strictness of lessons, but it is always fulfilling, and with the Grandness of truth.

The lesson of obedience is one of the harder lessons to learn, and that is why bat medicine can be controversial. Just about the time you think you've got it right, you find you were obedient to wrong. So is the bat evil or is it good? The bat is simply a bat—it just is. To be obedient is to realize that it is a bat and learn all about it. It seems evil, because it is a nocturnal animal, coming, therefore, from the dark. We always think that evil is dark. Maybe we should be obedient to truth and understand that evil is transparent. It can take on any color—it is black, it is white, and it is within Choice.

Aho.

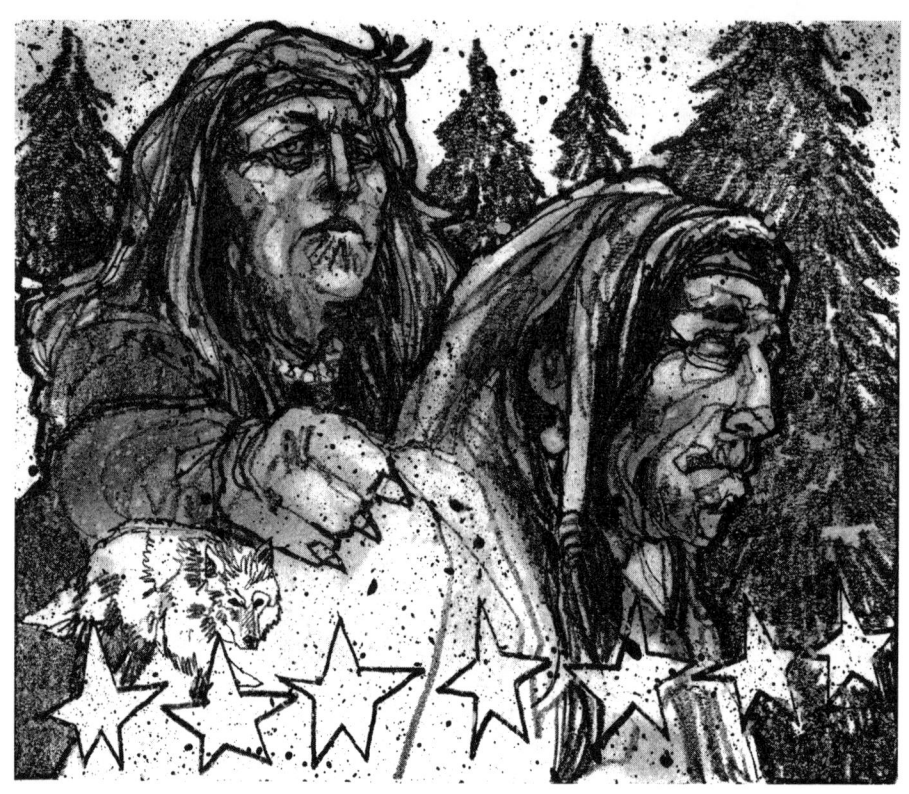

5

THE WIND'S VOICE— CEREMONY

It is dark, and candles are twinkling all around me. I stand in the center of the Medicine Wheel holding onto my faith. I came to Ceremony as a child. Once, when I was in a high fever and close to death with the chicken pox, weak and alone, I prayed, "Is anybody out there? Can anybody hear me? I'm a little girl, all alone." Yeah, I had people to take care of me; I had a couple who watched over me and they were wonderful German people—a kind and loving mom and dad. That doesn't change the fact that I was abandoned, that everybody was too busy— everybody being Mom and Dad.

I look up and my older sister is right in front of me.

"Hey, Mag. It's good to see you." I look around and there is a soft vapor of swirling yellow smoke all around. My sister has beautiful green eyes, soft skin, and pretty reddish-blond hair. She holds out her hand and on top of it is a ladybug.

"It's good to see you again, Maggie. That's one thing I like about the spirit world—I like seeing relatives. I like that about shamanism—I can connect with you people. I've got a lot of questions to ask. Do you remember when we were young and you told me to do a path map and I could lay out my life and everything could go just like I want it to? Well, I'm at that spot where I'm starting to wonder, when does it start to go like I want it to? Can you answer that question for me?"

She sits there quiet, with her legs crossed in her pedal pushers, her painted toenails, her one earring and her pixie hair cut.

"Man, Sis, you were always different. You were just always so different. It's so good to see you! Creativity follows you everywhere."

She just keeps looking at me, saying nothing. I hear a hollow wind sound, like angels singing, or the quiet whispering of the wind in winter. I lean forward a little. It sounds and feels very empty.

She reaches out her hand a little further, and the ladybug is crawling across it.

"Don't you have time to answer those questions?"

She looks at the ladybug. So I guess she wants me to take it. I reach out to get the ladybug and it flies away. I watch it, and it lands on a piece of grass. I start to get it.

"Hey, Maggie, was death as easy as you said it would be? I was wondering what happened because you fought so hard just before you died. You know, cancer is really unfair."

I reach for the ladybug and it flies away, outside the Medicine Wheel. I look back at my sister; she is no longer there, but I can hear her soft voice in the hollow sounds of the wind.

"Do you understand?" she says.

A quietness has come into her voice, and the voice of the wind is all there, whistling around me—deep, soft, and firm. Do I understand? I breathe in and out.

"I don't know if I understand sometimes. I have people coming tonight who want to have answers. They think they can wave a magic wand and things will change. I don't think I do understand any more

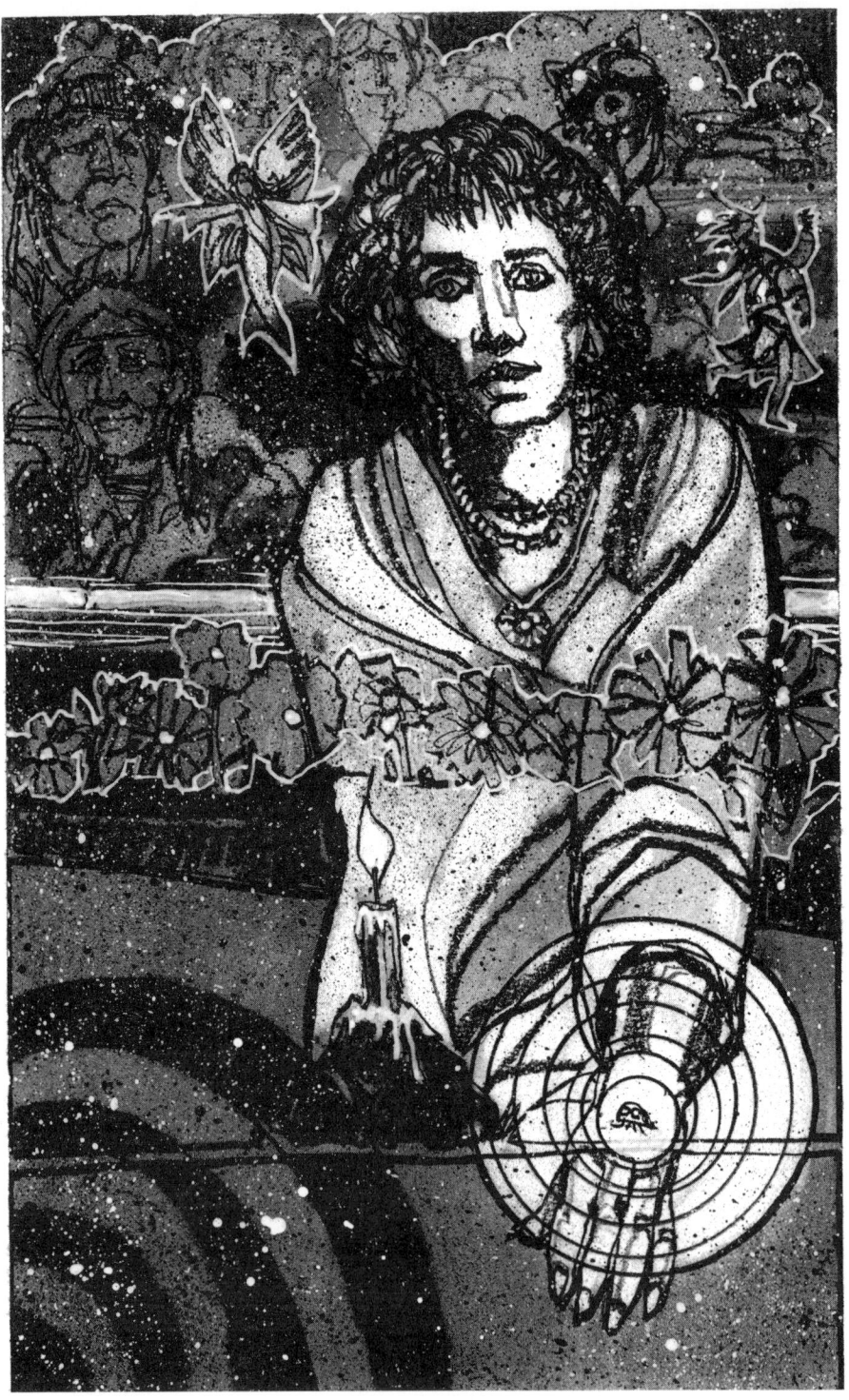

than what the Medicine Wheel has taught me, and now, Mom, you're gone, and Margaret, you're bringing me ladybugs. I don't know—sometimes the spirit world is really, really..."

"Really what, Wolf?" the old voice says.

I look to the West Gate and there stands Old Woman Rock. "Really what? Really mysterious? Really magical? Really what?"

"Oh, I guess I just want to turn to the South and curl up in my emotions and let the trickster, King Coyote, the Guardian of the South, kick me around a little."

"Go ahead. Head on back to your emotions. Walk forward around the Medicine Wheel and walk right back into them, for they are there for you to feel and that's what you're doing right now. You've got a lot of feelings, girl, and you've still got a long way to go around the wheel."

"Hey, did you see that ladybug?"

"Oh, yeah, I know that ladybug. I know that bug. It carries with it the opportunity of Ceremony. Right after Choice the energy swirls," and she moves her hand around clockwise." It swirls, and with all of its yellow frequency it brings about its creativity." She looks at me with a twinkle in her eyes. "You know, that's the voice of your vision. The wind's voices—they are all our opportunities," and she continues to move her hand clockwise around the wheel. "You see, Wolf, you must understand purpose. You must remember."

"Oh, I know," I say. "I need to remember my parents." I lean back and put both my hands on the ground, take a big deep breath and look up into the night sky. "Wow, there are no stars tonight. It's just dark."

"No, Wolf, not your parents. You know your parents. Can you tell me you know your parents?"

"Yes, it's the sun and the moon. My parents are life and death. My parents were physical—a male and a female—but they were life and death."

I feel my face become stone. My body is sinking hard into the ground. My heart is beating fast; ever since those chicken pox, my life has been running out—the abuse of physical existence, trying to stay away from the memories of pain. How can anyone be so brutal and hurt a child so badly? I turn and look at Old Woman as she stands there. She has cloaked herself and wrapped her blanket tight around her.

"I am rejecting those thoughts, Wolf, for I am in balance, for I am rock, and rock is total solidity. Those are your emotions."

"Yeah, I know that. They're my emotions, they're mine, and all I want to do is have somebody feel sorry for me, cloak me in their robe and carry me off into their life."

"You have the answers. They have been given to you from Great Spirit, Grandmother/Grandfather. Through your Grandmother and Grandfather Wolf you can learn. You can rise above the pain, as you tell your students. It is your Choice. Remember what you say to them?" she says with intensity in her voice. I cannot see her face, it is covered with her blanket.

"Yeah, I remember what I say to them, and I know it's true, 'cause every step I take within the Rainbow Medicine Wheel opens the opportunities for me."

"Where do you think that ladybug went?"

"It went outside the wheel. That's a funny thing, too. I get up and walk over to the East gate and leave this wheel—and I am no longer in the medicine wheel, but yet I'm still in the medicine wheel. I say that to my students, you know, Old Woman, and they look at me like I've lost my mind."

"That's because we get limited," she says. "That's the hard thing about symbols like crosses, and titles like schools, and places we go to. We get limited and we get shut way down." She points at the yellow rock. "The third medicine stone in the West section of the wheel—this is Ceremony." She points at the third rock in the lesson stones of the West section of the wheel. "This is life. Who is your sister again?" she asks me.

"My sister? She was a gypsy, she was a wandering wildflower. My Mom named her Wildflower. We laughed at that one time when we were young, 'cause Maggie said, 'Yeah, I'm a wildflower, I like to wander from here to there,' and she did, too. There was never a wine bottle that wasn't her friend. There was never a home that she wasn't a family member of. She blew through the air like a wildflower seed."

"Who was your sister, again?" Old Woman says.

"Oh, I love you people in spirit world. You just keep on until I say what you want me to, don't you?"

"No. No," Old Woman Rock replies. "We just keep talking until it comes to pass that you understand the rock you're now embarking upon."

"My sister? She was a human being."

"Do you understand?" I hear her say.

I look at Old Woman Rock cloaked in her blanket. "Are you my sister, Old Woman Rock? Is that why I can't see your face?"

"No, no, no, I'm only a human being." She looks at me, closes her eyes slowly, and then opens them. "The only point in physicality is that we understand we are human beings."

Everything in front of me becomes a rainbow. Swirling shades of reds and oranges, yellows and greens, blues and purples—soft mist engulfs me.

"We're limited on Earth to race, to family, to places. Some of us are chained down by what we make for a living. Humans are free to live like the ladybug," Old Woman says.

The ladybug lands on the Creator rock and the candle at the center flickers.

"I remember a Ceremony that my sister taught me once," I say. "It was prayer, and we were praying with a white candle, and the candle went way down low—the flame did—and almost went out." I watch the candle flickering in front of me, as I tell this story. "We prayed. We were praying for a good friend of mine who had died. The candle went out and I reached forward to light it again and my sister said, "No," and just as she did, the flame of the candle flipped back on and grew large again.

She says, "Remember this. You'll know when I am present when I am a spirit. You'll always know that spirit is present when the candle flame goes almost out, or goes out, and comes back on again. You'll know that we are listening and that we are present—all of us, all spirit beings."

I look over Old Woman's head above the medicine wheel and the sky is full of billowing clouds, all in color. They have circled us. There are faces in the clouds, and angels with large wings. I look another way, and there are kachinas and dancers from the Southwest. I look another way and see animal spirits, dancers from the Circle of Life. I look another way, and there are plant and flower spirits, animals spirits, and people's faces that I recognize—my Momma Till, my Granny Lil, all the old ones there in the sky.

"Oh, that's not sky, Wolf. That's real. You forgot where you are."

"Wow, Old Woman, the spirits are so big."

"That's because you are still a human and you are so small."

It's a wonderful feeling watching all these spirits move around me. I sit, quietly, watching the flame of the candle flicker.

"That Ceremony was true, Old Woman," I say, and she is gone.

The river flows softly by. Home. I am home, for a moment again. Wow. The smells—the smells of Fall along the river, the cottonwood, the oak—the beautiful blanket of colors that line the hillsides. I feel excitement in my heart. If this is home and that's the river, he must be here. I can smell the river flock, a purple flower that grows wild by the river bank. Its mysterious sweet smell is always around when he is there.

My mind drifts to his dark eyes, to his youth, to his strong chest.

I see him run across the river, dancing across the stones, standing on the other side.

"Catch me if you can, Wolf. Come on, run with me."

I stand up to chase him, and as I begin to run I realize it is a Ceremony. I move across the rocks, agile and swift, and catch up with him. He is standing there, slow and tired. He is mature, fully mature—past fifty—white in his hair. He slings it around and shakes the water off, just as he did when we were young.

"Life's a Ceremony, Wolf, and everything in it is just a circle."

I watch him move towards his camp with a limp, walking slow.

"Do you get old and die?"

"Look at yourself in the water," he says.

I look, and there is white hair along my temples.

"The White Wolf comes forth. It won't be long now until snow medicine will be all that you are. They tell me you're searching out Ceremony. Our relationship has been a Ceremony from beginning to end."

He grabs a cloth and is drying his head and shaking his hair around like a wild animal, strong in stature, even though old in years. I still feel the intensity in those dark eyes. His beard is sprinkled with white, but his skin is still golden.

"We are the two-legged. We are humans. That is the grandest Ceremony of all, and we have lived it."

"Granddaughter!" echoes out across the river. "Get up here, Granddaughter."

"I have to go. Grandmother Wolf calls." I spin and fly, my feet barely touching the ground. Coming into home, sitting on the porch in Fall, is truly Ceremony.

"Granddaughter, we have some news. We have things for you to do. You must prepare to listen to the story of the bones. You must get ready and gather your medicine."

"Grandmother, have I got any time so I can go back and see Dark Eyes for a moment? I can't believe he's getting old."

"Granddaughter," Grandmother Wolf says with a smile in her old wrinkled face, "Dark Eyes never gets old. Be careful. Don't you know he is simply playing upon your pity? He's not old. He's alive and young. Nothing in Ceremony, nothing in spirit ever gets old. It is only in your physical existence, when you are calling upon the truths, when you are trying to understand the wind's voice, that you feel any part of age. It is when you are seeking."

"But Grandmother, you look old."

"No, I look wise. Each line is a story. Each moment brought down the sag in my face. Wise is not old. There is a long way beyond wrinkling. Old is smooth. Old is so smooth that when it's wet in the river you slide off and bump your butt. Don't you know the story of a rock?" she says.

The wind dances through the cottonwood trees and the fire smells of burning oak drift across my nose, and I can smell home—the smell of leather, food cooking, and fresh flowers, sweet and soft.

"Yep, that's right. You can. But there is no river flock, Granddaughter, it's Fall."

"What do you mean there's no river flock? I could smell it."

"No. You could smell him, his essence, the essence of romance, the essence of passion—things that will get you in trouble, Granddaughter. Now I want you to get inside right now," and she grabs me by the ear. In the door she pushes me, and right down in front of the altar I go—kerplunk. "Now you get your things together, and you wrap your medicine bundle, 'cause you're off to see Snake Man, and he will speak to you of his vision. You must understand change. You must understand that you will be confronted by Choice one more time, and it will be the Choice of your heart. It will take you into the adventure of your mind. It will be long after this moment, through the doors of Impeccable, and on past the impeccable teachings in the Song, that you will understand. But there will come a moment soon, when Grandfather and I can no longer tell you stories. You will be grown. It will be time to live in balance, and there can be no hate, no anger, no anguish. No unbalanced emotions, in other words. Do you understand me?"

"Yes, Grandmother," I say, in a childish, girlish voice. Boy, I don't understand her. I try hard when I'm on Earth to put this all together. I sit there with my eagle feather in front of me, listening—listening and trying to figure it all out.

I look on the floor, where a ladybug is crawling along.

I hear the rattling of the bones calling me back.

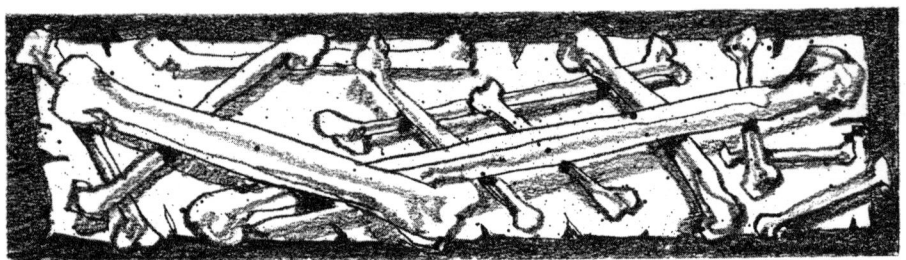

Teachings of Ceremony—Ladybug Medicine

Ceremony is one of the most exciting acts that a human can participate in, for it is a circle. It is one of many sacred circles in life. You can see the movement of the circle of Ceremony in human existence—we are born, we grow, we mature, we age, we die. When you work within Ceremony, you begin to realize that everything you do in life is a Ceremony. You sleep, you eat, you reproduce, you even play because you start and finish. In other words, you start at a spot and come back to the same spot. That movement is the movement of Ceremony.

Ceremony should not be confused with worship or religion. I think there are four elements that come together, which I like to call "action elements," that produce a healthy life. They are to be spiritual, to be religious, to worship, and to do Ceremony. Spiritual and Ceremony go together, and worship and religion go together, because you can have Ceremony without religion, but you can't have worship without religion. So spiritually, life is a Ceremony and religiously, life is worship. A lot of people see religion and worship as Ceremony and spiritual, and that is because spiritual and Ceremony come before all things, and all things come from, and are, spiritual Ceremony.

The totem of Ceremony is the ladybug. Her body is round, there is color to her; she takes flight, and she brings joy to people. Therefore, she reveals herself as a Ceremony—from stillness to flight to stillness, the ladybug's life goes on.

The teachings of Ceremony are:

1. Strict. The key to success is the confidence and strength that a Ceremony has. That can be seen in its strictness—the timing, the clothing, the objects used in the Ceremony, and the words and songs spoken and sung. They have to be the way they always are, the way they were written to be, for the Ceremony to be performed.

2. Respect. When performing a Ceremony, there comes a balance that brings about success. This balance comes from respect. When you are taught to perform Ceremony, there must be a common ground of respect, so that everyone joined together will receive, and everyone joined together will be enlightened. Respecting people's rights, respecting their race, respecting their beliefs, contributes to the success of a Ceremony.

3. Color. Color in a Ceremony is the vital heartbeat. Color is the movement of Change, as in the Ceremony of life from one season to the next. The beautiful Changes that go on through a year are the Ceremony of the year's life.

4. The Elements. Elements are necessary for there to be a physical action that we call Ceremony. Elements such as water, fire, air, earth, rain, snow, food, opening, closure—each element brings forth the totality of a Ceremony.

5. Solemn. Being solemn within Ceremony brings about the profound, the holy, the serious, the earnest actions needed to receive, transmit, understand, and live a Ceremony. What I mean by that is, when we take things for granted, we soon forget that they are Ceremony. Often a marriage Ceremony is taken for granted and the marriage ends in divorce. But if it is profound, magical, special, solemn, earnest, it very well may last way into fifty and more years.

6. Politeness. Politeness within Ceremony is never to cross anybody's boundaries, spiritually or physically. Crossing boundaries is to name-call, to blaspheme, to mock, to be haughty, to be selfish, and it is one of the hardest movements of Ceremony. Respect makes politeness easy.

You need to join hands for there to be a perfect Ceremony. If you are performing a Ceremony by yourself, you need to lift your hands to the sky with your palms open to the stars. You are holding hands, then, with the stars.

7. Sacred. To set apart from and to make special is what sacred feels like within a proper Ceremony. Not taking it for granted or believing that it is the same as everything else. Sacred sets apart and lifts above. What I mean by that is to expect a miracle in every Ceremony. To expect magic and success. Sacred is applying knowledge, tradition, and festivity with respect and politeness, knowing what to feed the earth, how to make it smell, what colors are necessary for vibration frequencies—all these techniques come together in sacredness in a Ceremony. To perform a Ceremony, the only thing you need is an honest heart, heart being very much the mind.

Simple things in life like combing your hair, eating breakfast, exercising, raising your children, working, and praying, are Ceremony. All things in life are Ceremony. But a ceremonialist performs Ceremony in a public way to bring about actions such as a marriage, a funeral, the blessing of a child, the blessing of a home. To perform these actions, it is necessary to know the difference between action and Ceremony. Before anyone calls herself or himself a ceremonialist, my personal advice is to study Ceremony from an appropriate ceremonial teacher.

I wish that everyone who sets out to perform Ceremony will succeed and be happy. Every moment of your life is the Ceremony that Great Spirit has given us that we call our human physical existence.

Aho.

Ceremonial Stick

TOOLS: *A stick four to seven feet tall (1.2 to 2.1m); four large feathers—red, green, blue, and white; seven smaller feathers, one each red, orange, yellow, green, blue, purple, and burgundy; a strip of red 100% cotton cloth 24 inches long by half an inch wide (60 x 1.25cm); a strip of blue 100% cotton cloth 24 inches long by one-and-a-half inches wide (60 x 2cm); colored string or embroidery thread; fifty-six jingle bells, yellow waterproof paint, smudge bowl, fan, and herbs.*

For a ceremonial stick, find one that represents your dedication to Ceremony. The stick should be four to seven feet tall and not any bigger around than your arm. When you are collecting your feathers, they can be any type that fits the Ceremony that you carry in your heart. I recommend turkey feathers or the pre-dyed white ones that you can find in your local crafts store. The feathers represent the medicines and the lessons that are within the Ceremony of your life. The four large feathers should be either painted or marked red, green, blue, and white. The others should be all the colors—red, orange, yellow, green, blue, purple, and burgundy. If you want, you can paint the edges of the feathers, or simply wrap embroidery thread around the end of the feather shaft, using the color of the feather needed for the Ceremony.

To make your ceremonial stick, first perform the Sacred Ceremony of Sacred Herbs: Smudge everything that you are going to use and balance yourself.

Vision things that your stick will represent when it is standing at your medicine wheel, such as ceremonies you will perform with it, prayers you will pray, dances you will learn. Write in your journal what you will do while holding your Ceremonial Stick.

Example: *Weddings, namings, weather dances, vision quests.*

Begin by wrapping the stick at the top with your favorite color. Then add the color of your spirit—the color that you think your spirit is. Then add your clan color—the color that you designate as your family

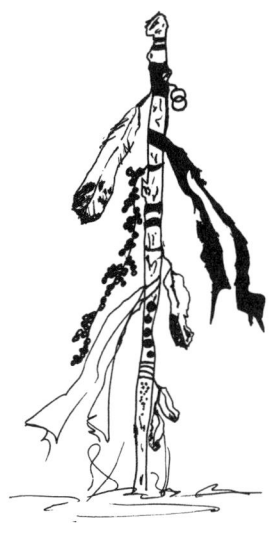

color or a traditional color that has been brought about by your family. Then if you have nation colors, wrap the pole with those.

After you have completed that, tie the red and blue cloths onto the stick to represent the Red Road and the Blue Road of the Medicine Wheel. Then tie the fifty-six bells in long strands to jingle on the pole to represent the medicines and the lessons going out into your life. Each time you hear the bells, or rattle or touch the bells, remember that you are in balance with your lessons in Rainbow Medicine, that you are walking with the medicines in Rainbow Medicine.

Take the yellow paint and paint the stick the way you see fit for your Ceremony—stripes, solid, polka dots, spirals. Painting the yellow onto the stick represents your creativity, your vision, your Ceremony, and your prayer.

When you have finished your stick, sharpen the end that is to go in the ground. Place the pole outside at your Medicine Wheel, or outside your home in the ground, or leaning against your door. This is your ceremonial pole to be used any time that you perform Ceremony. You can hold this pole in your hands or stand at this pole and do prayers when you need to change things in your life—like eating better, dieting, getting more rest, studying harder, or becoming a better person. You can sit at this pole and do prayers; you can carry this pole and go on long walks and think about what you should be doing to achieve the ceremonies that you set out to do.

When your ceremonial pole starts to look worn and weathered, it is a good thing, for it is taking on the medicine of weather, achievement, and age. Age, weathering, wrinkling, crumpling, and fading are signs the medicine is strong in this stick. You can touch up the pole any time you want to, making it fresh by simply adding new paint or new symbols. Never take away the old, always add to it. The old is medicine (memories).

Aho.

Ceremony of Light

TOOLS: *Cornmeal, candles of all colors—twelve or more; candleholder for each candle; pen and journal; medicine blanket; smudge bowl, fan, and herbs.*

Find a place in which you can build a cornmeal circle where you won't be disturbed. If you are going to do the Ceremony outside, wet the ground down first to make sure the candles won't catch the ground or grass on fire. If you are going to do the Ceremony inside, use candleholders and take all precautions so as not to have any type of fire hazard or accident in your home. When you have found the place where the Ceremony will be done, place cornmeal, tobacco, or sage on the ground as a give-away to the four-legged and the spirits, the crawlies, and anyone else who comes.

Set up the candles by putting them in their candleholders and placing them where you wish them to go—at your altar, on the floor in front of you, or around the center of the medicine wheel. Each candle represents a thought—something you worry about, something you need to pray for, something you want to have, something you have had, a good deed you wish for, anything and everything that prayers are for you. Place candles for loved ones and others that you want to pray for.

As you set your candles, make your prayers. White candles can be used for any and all things. Colored candles are to be connected to your medicine and lesson words. When you are praying for things that are from the physical body, I suggest you use blue. When you are praying for wholeness, I suggest you use black. When you are praying for protection and safety, I suggest turquoise; for spiritual matters I suggest silver or white, and for matters of money and finance, gold.

When you light your candles, take out your journal, sit on your medicine blanket, and take your time watching the candles burn, letting go of all fear and balancing such emotions as sadness and anger. Remember that being happy and joyful is just as stressful as being sad and fearful. Come to a place within yourself that is very quiet within prayer. Journal any feelings that you might have from the Ceremony or things you want to remember that come to you while visioning and listening, watching and feeling the Ceremony of Light.

Enjoy the beauty of the Ceremony of Light and relax. When you light the candles, try to remember which way you lit them and which ones you lit first. When you are closing your Ceremony, you can move counterclockwise, snuffing the candles with your fingers. Snuff out the ones you lit last, first.

When you are through with your Ceremony, conduct the Ceremony of the Sacred Herbs, smudging the area and letting go of the situation, moving back into your life. Put everything away and leave your sacred Ceremony of Light for any time you wish to come and sit and be in the presence of the Ceremony. Do not leave the Ceremony unattended and burning without being there. You can burn the candles until they are completely gone and then replace them, letting the wax build up from the old candles that have been in the Ceremony.

If the day should come when you choose not to have a Ceremony of Light altar or space, dig a hole in the earth and dismiss it by burning all the candle wax and the memories of the Ceremony, covering it over and offering tobacco, cornmeal, and sacred herbs to the ground. I suggest you put no metal or wire from the candles in the ground—dispose of them in a proper way.

Aho.

Process of the Lesson of Life—Teachings of the Human Being

The process of the lesson of life is something that each of us as human beings—two-legged, mankind, womankind—have to experience when we are brought to life through reproduction. Creation figures into our human existence. Our physical existence looks like it is separated and lonely from Great Spirit, for it gets sick, it breaks down, it dies. But in fact what it is, is even closer to Great Spirit than anyone can imagine, for it is the most precious thing that Great Spirit has created. We as human two-leggeds take our lives for granted. We drift away from life. Even though we live every day, many of us are empty and lifeless.

To experience and understand the lessons of life, we must travel through what I call the Sacred Circle of Physical Existence:

1. Animation. The circle starts with liveliness, spirit. It is hard to find words that express clearly the power of spirit. So often we are separated from spirit, which is animation. The best word I have found to describe the perpetual, constant vast experience of what we call God, Creator, Great Spirit, Jehovah, is animation, for it is exaggerated, expressive, colorful, and energetic—all the words that life, as we know it, is. First, before mankind, was a being. Animation, which is spirit, existed, and from that animation comes our existence.

2. Existence. Color, vigor, vastness, energy. Existence is your spirit. To grasp the concept of life, it is essential to see it as a spiral with no beginning and no end. Your personal spirit comes forth long before you come to this earth. Your spirit often is the thought that brings your parents together, that motivates them to reproduce. Your spirit lives long before its physical existence.

3. Enliven. Vigorous, active, bright, and energetic, it is your soul, your spiritual silver connection with Great Spirit that is never broken. We often feel that we are detached from God, that maybe we're not good enough, not ready, or maybe we've committed sins and we're separated from Great Spirit, God, Creator. Enliven is the energy point, the moment that we reconnect through our soul, the pathway connection of energy with Great Spirit.

4. Resilience. Our spiritual essence, it is our temperature from spirit—hot and cold—that in the long run brings about our body temperature, an equal balance regulated by physical parts of our body. The resilience in our lives is our ability to recover. It comes from electric magnetic energy. It takes the four processes of heat and cold, electric and magnetic, to bring us into form.

5. Being. It is the shape that our aura—energy field—takes on. It is the movement through the sacred tunnels of energy called chakras, which give us our form. This form is often much larger than just our physical form. Our form may sometimes be very small and quiet, in the very core of our mind—that which we call our heart.

6. Reproduction. Body. When we are created, we are cycled energy brought forth into mass, known as matter. Life is a mystery, yet every day it becomes more and more understood. Our bodies are made up of the sacred movements of physicality, which are breath, heartbeat, feelings, and thought. When we choose to reproduce, these four elements bring forth the spirit of the child. The life force in these elements is revealed in the complex movements of our physical bodies. We pass our essence on through our children.

7. Force. Our vitality, our exuberance, our destinies, and our fates, our faith, our spirituality, our Ceremony. It is the final step, which is death, that takes us back into pure animation, pure spirit.

Life draws its energy from spirit. There are no human words big enough, bright enough, or energetic enough to describe the spirit of Great Spirit. The human language is limited. To explain spirit, see me hold my arms straight out and everything outside of my arms is spirit. I have to quote a student who once said, "Mystery is the great what is." And that, simply put by another student, is "all."

Aho.

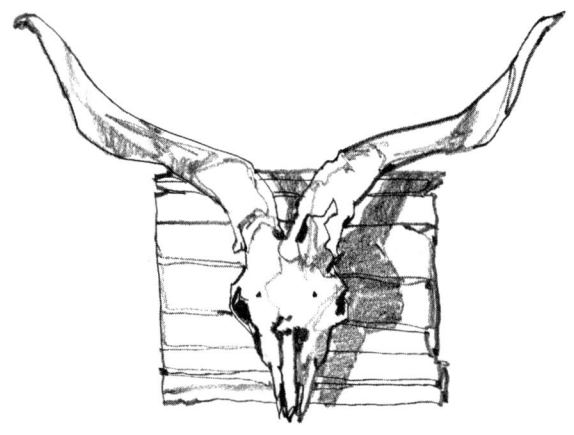

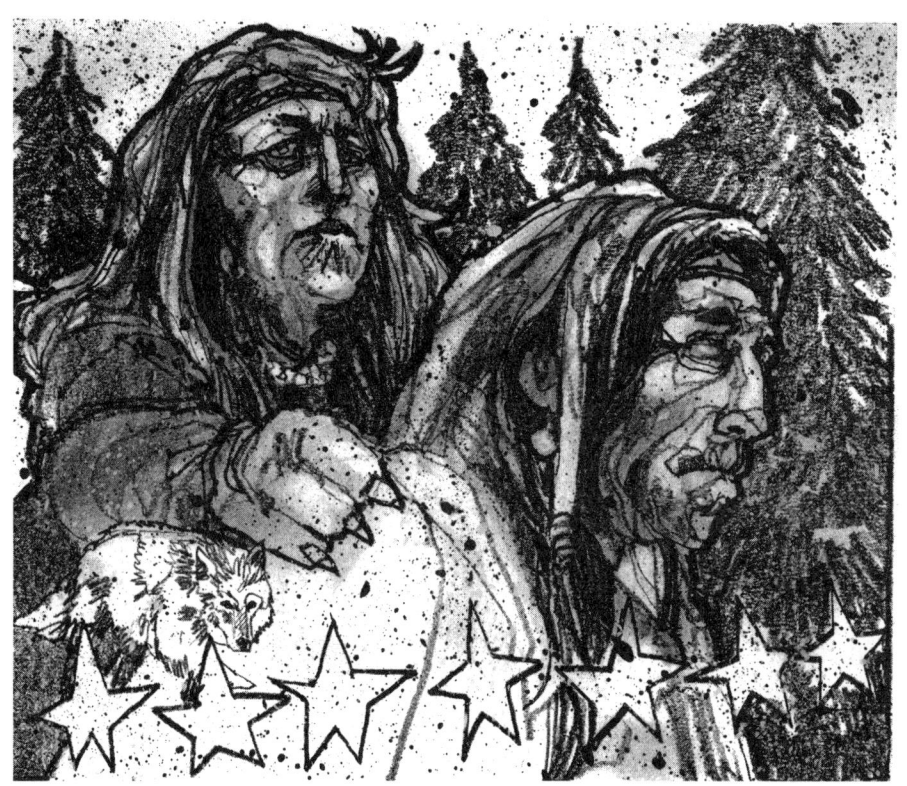

6
SNAKE MAN'S VISION— CHANGE

I breathe in and out, and I relax. Everything around me is green. Beautiful green grass, all types of green trees—aspens and apples, pines and cedars, every kind of tree and plant and bush. They are flowering and they smell so strong. I breathe in and out. Walking along this magnificent path, I look out at the mountains' splendor. They are etched with snow, a light Fall dusting.

E.G. is right. Obedience is the lesson that carries you into understanding. Without obedience and reverence and respect, I would not be able to even begin to understand the lessons of life.

"That's right. That's right," a voice says. "Many, many do not know.

They only think."

I look and there stands the one I know as Snake Man, with his long silver braids, his snake eyes, and his black hat dusty with age. One hand is in his pocket, the other holds his walking stick. His shirt, the familiar calico pattern, is burgundy with yellow stars. A bandanna is tied around his neck; a snake head makes up his belt buckle; and his boots are snakeskin. He wears a very large knife on his belt, and a necklace of snake vertebrae hangs down the front of his shirt in several layers, with rattlesnake tails.

"Boy, I sure would like to hug you," I hear myself saying. "I feel I have always known you. You remind me of home."

"Oh," he says, with a warm, welcoming smile. "There in your time you could touch. That's a good thing about being a human. Here—feel—me. That's touch."

I take a breath. I need to ground myself. I feel faint.

"Walk," he says. "Let's go to camp." So we take a long walk. He is silent. The morning is warm and rich.

"Nothing like a walk on a Fall morning," I say.

No answer from him. We come into camp and there is his fire, and beside it the stump where he sits, and a blanket on the ground partially covering another stump.

"Sit there. I want to show you something."

So we sit down, and he says, "Look." He points at the fire pit. It is a circle with circles inside it, with lines coming out that make it look like a spider web. In the center there is a herkimer crystal the size of my fist that shimmers in the morning light. Around that stone a circle of beautiful stars, all different colors, is twinkling and glittering.

I feel the warm sun on my face and I smell the fresh air, the crisp pines, the earth aromas all around me. I am sitting in a circle of Ceremony, a medicine wheel that I am part of. A woman is approaching me and she hands me a rock with a snake on it.

"Listen to her," Snake Man says.

I listen very carefully and hear soft rattling. Soon there is also a clicking, and the rattling gets louder. The stars are pulsating.

"These stars you see are the Bone People." Snake Man looks at me with his eyes closed, his nose almost touching his chin, nodding ever so gently. "These are lives, coming here through the web of life, coming here." He nods.

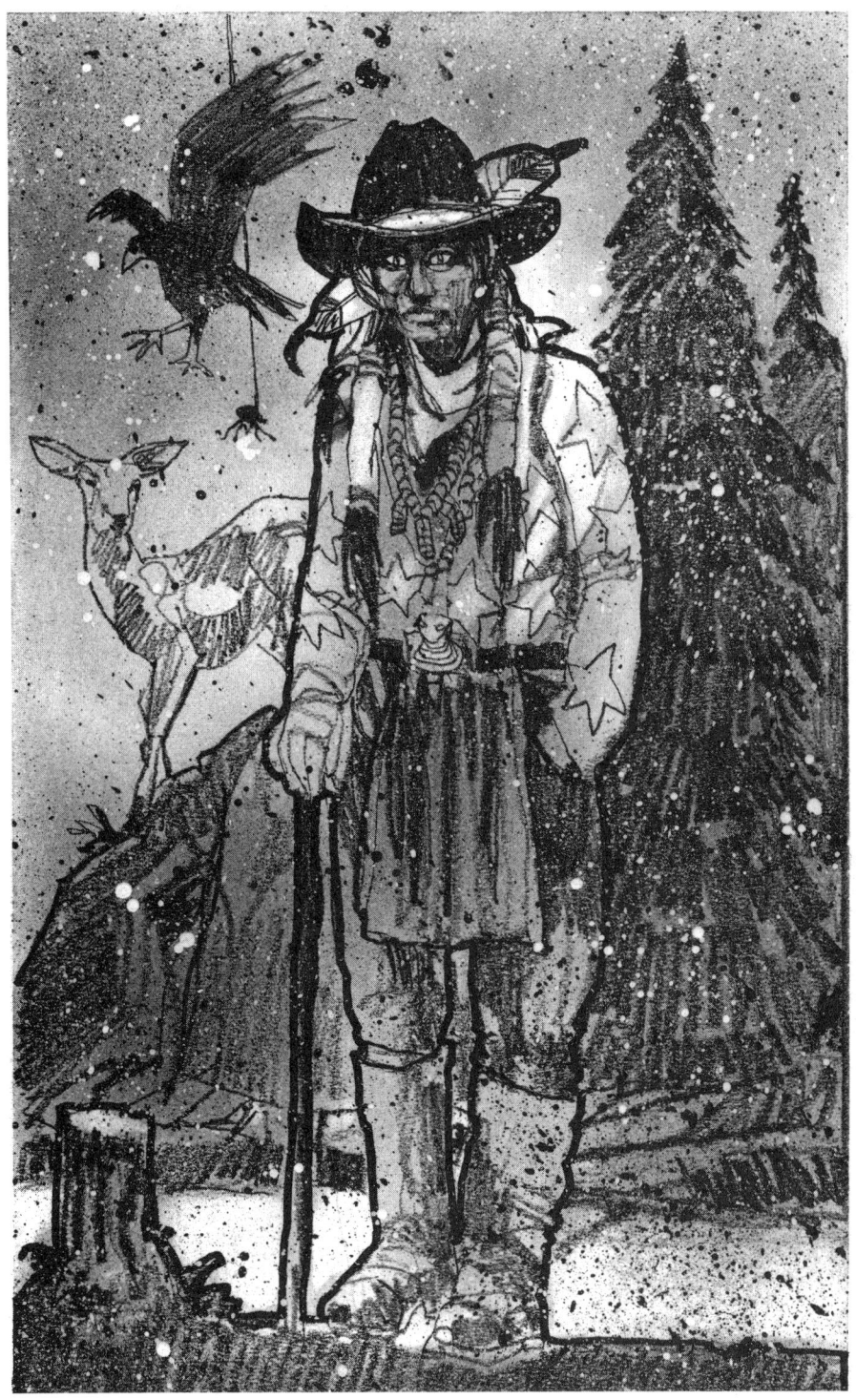

The bone people, star people, spiral around the center of the wheel like dewdrops on a spider web. The bone people work their way out in circles, getting bigger and bigger. I can hear the rattling of bones.

"Look close."

I can see people—many people. All colors of people. Behind me I can hear the soft gentle movement of water, the creek that rolls along, a familiar, relaxing sound. As the stars get to the edges of the circles, they burst forth and scatter into the air. They are all around me, darting off, bouncing, sparkling in the trees.

"You see, life is perpetually coming and going, like Change. Once, a long time ago, a very tiny green spirit was born and it grew into Change. It had a twin named Chance. Before they were born, there was no movement. There was nothing but still. They emerged from Ceremony, which was a Choice of Nurture, and Great Spirit said there would be life. He Nurtured, he loved, he created. A Choice to experience, to have opportunity, emerged through the ceremony of connection to reality. Life is ever-moving Change/Chance. Stillness opens the door to Ceremony. A Ceremony is Choice. Great Spirit brought all forth from the Ceremony of Choice. There stand these twins, two green—one Change, one Chance. They move out and bring Proof of Great Spirit's love. Real, the purple spirit, stands. It steps out of its coldness into life. Grand life."

He opens his eyes, and they twinkle at me with a depth of knowledge—the snake eyes, the deep eyes of knowing.

"Don't you think that everyone would hate a snake for knowing the truth? Don't you think that if there is evil, it would be hating a snake?" he says. "I know that we are given Change in life, and that's the only way we have chance. If something's not good, then just throw it in the fire—Change—bury it, forget it. Change. Buy a new one, get rid of it. Change. Tear it down, build it up. Change. Nothing in life moves without Change, and there is no life without Change—there is nothing without Change."

He stands there shaking his head, wobbling left and right. The sun dances off his cheekbones and the wind softly blows the afternoon towards us.

"I will leave you now, with this vision in your mind," and he puts his fingers on his forehead and pushes his hand down straight with two fingers pointing at the vision. "Look," he says quickly.

I look at the vision, but there is nothing there but a fire pit.

"There! That is Ceremony. Now you have a Choice. Always remember, when the emotions are sad, choose happy. When filled with fear, choose acceptance. Always a Choice," he says. "Someone waits for you in the woods. Someone who holds great Change in your life. You will soon embrace the vision. Remember the twins—Change and Chance."

I find myself walking in the woods, looking at the lush ferns and thinking about the depth of life beneath my feet. I can smell the river ahead. I don't have a care in the world, I am free. I am looking forward, walking, when all of a sudden in front of me is the most beautiful woman I have ever seen. She has beautiful reddish-chestnut hair. Her eyes are soft brown, and she stands in her kindness and softness, waving her hand back and forth. Then I see a deer—a doe she is—shifting and changing from deer to two-legged. A soft green mist floats around her. I can see stars, tiny ones with laughter like children. Many children's voices sing and laugh around her. She fades from deer to woman. She is Fading Deer.

"Hi, Wolf. Listen. This is hard for me to say to you. You must pay attention, for you will bring grief and sadness to the elders if you don't listen to my message. You must move on. Change has come for you. The Wind of Change brings life. Within the forest it is the very home and beginning of all who emerge into human and four-legged form. All that we are here, is birth through Change. Each of us has our chance."

Her deer tail twitches as she speaks. Fading Deer is soft and gentle, with big brown eyes. "There is another," she says with fear. "Beware of Deer Woman."

Fading Deer disappears in the woods. There is late morning dew glittering on the limbs of the trees, and I watch a spider build its web. Every process is Change.

The spider looks at me and asks, "Do you recognize me? I am Change. You will know me by the fear, for I am scared of myself."

I look carefully at the spider. It is black. It is deadly—a black widow.

"That's right. Everyone is afraid of me, for I am chance. Take a chance and let me bite you. Will you live?"

"I choose not to be bit," I say.

"That's a wise choice for I am the most treacherous of all medicine, the arrow of truth—a blue arrow. Beware of the white arrow, for it pierces your heart. Truth does not pierce: it is carried. It is honor and integrity, and visions of Dark Eyes are simply loneliness and emptiness. They are the foreboding of destruction."

I watch the spider weave its way around its silver core, building its web, speaking truths as it works its intricate designs with its legs and feet. The sun glimmers rainbows within the web.

"Yes, it is easy to mistake me for the rainbow maker. I am no rainbow maker. I am the one they speak of as deadly, but I am simply survival. You speak with E.G. of how evil the wolf and bat and raven are. That is what mankind says about them, that is true. They kill me—when I am only surviving to carry on my species. The chance for all mankind is in the secrets of Grand. Would you tear my web down for no reason? Would you smash me only because I'm ugly? Then it would be your Choice to create a Ceremony of death as an action of fear. Everything, Wolf, has a reason."

Her voice is soft and feminine. I watch her work; she is intriguing.

"You need not worry about what challenges your mind, for you have many chances. Never fear that you have only one. Never fear that Dark Eyes will be your last chance. You will be overcome by his poison and call it love. He is the emptiness of your mind. It is in your own mind, Wolf—the abandonment. He is nothing." Her eyes sparkle as she speaks. "Run from him, for this time is physical and your mind will become his! He will be your thoughts. You will think only him."

I look beyond her and there is the river rushing by, and on the other side the familiar Dark Eyes, standing in the morning sun, stretching and flexing, drawing in his magnificent beauty. I stand in the serene setting, watching the water rush by, bounding off the rocks. In the river are rocks of jasper, rocks of crystal, rocks of amethyst, emeralds, rubies, hematites, and herkimer—all stones. The river of stones. The water rushes quickly over the rocks.

I want to run to him and ask him if he knows about the last chance, ask him if he is real, for I know he can give me the answers, like he always has. I start to cross, when a woman appears. She is sleek and intense. She walks towards him. He waves for me to come. She reaches up, digs her nails into his shoulder, and hangs on. He pulls away from her and her fingernails leave marks on his skin. He drops to his knees in weakness and staggers. He is faint with age. He disappears.

I turn to leave, and there, standing in front of me, is the woman. She looks at me with piercing, cutting black eyes, sharp jawbones, the strong features of the deer.

She is brilliant, exquisite. Her hair is rich, chocolate brown. She is fresh and agile. Her humanness is dressed in the skin of a deer, a dress with long fringe on the left side. She wears a necklace of bones and stones. In the center of that necklace is white fur. Her nails are long, capable of...

"Digging deep into the soul," she says, as she smiles. She lifts her fingers, pointing her nails towards me. "Trade me him for the song. I will give you the secrets of the song. What is a wolf without its song! You know, 'Somewhere over the Rainbow,'" she laughs. "Your medicine is weak and you are weak."

She glares at me. I feel weak—I must overcome these thoughts.

"What is the matter, Wolf? Don't you like my song?

"I have nothing to trade—he's yours," I say.

She begins to sing. I walk off. I don't understand—this is not my song.

She seductively leans against the tree, throwing her head back. The sun sparkles off her radiant deep-set eyes. As she turns her head to the left, I see a hollowness, an ugliness, a thirst that cannot be quenched.

"Okay," she says. "You get what you want, I grant you that. But remember, I am the one he has chosen, for I enlighten him with my quickness and my agility. I am slender. I am all that beauty is."

Her words pierce my heart. He has chosen her? How is it that bitter, harsh, sharp feelings can burn so deep?

"Heh, heh," she laughs. "You have felt nothing yet," she laughs, cocking her head from right to left. "You spend all your time looking for answers and being intense. You're way too intense for me. You don't take time to laugh. You don't take time to enjoy. You need to lighten up—that's why you've lost."

I hear the caw of the raven. I look over her head and see a large raven circling us.

"How can you lose something you never chose?" I say. "What have I had—a few dances in the moonlight with him? Chasing him constantly to learn the secrets this wild man across the river has. I never chose. I lose nothing."

"Oh, you lose!" She circles me. "I want you to lose. I want you to feel Change. I want you to emerge and challenge me. I want you to fight me. I want to be your last chance. I want to own your very soul. I want you eaten up with jealousy. I want you to understand ownership. I want you to realize that woman owns man. They are bound together forever, pledging their love. Entangled, twisted, engulfed in passion," she says, stretching her beautiful, long neck, her beautiful legs. She is powerful in her intensity.

"I guess you don't like me, do you?"

"This isn't about 'like.' I have a purpose. I am about ownership." She lifts an eyebrow, points her finger at my heart, and says, "You lose."

I can't help but think of E.G. and the cave. Am I still in purpose, I wonder? What is the purpose of Change and chance? I must know the song of my vision.

She calls to me, "Give me his soul! I own him! He is mine!"

"How can you take love apart? I have chosen to follow his dance in the moonlight because he asked me to. His spirit dances at the river, a place I know as home. It seems that we are one circle, you and I."

She smiles. "You and I are *not!*"

I turn away and walk a few steps. "Is that all there is to this story? Is that all there is?"

I hear the caw of the raven. "No, there is your vision," the raven says. "You must sing the joy of your spirit. There are those who listen."

I turn and the one who taunted and tested me is gone. But there in the sky is a rainbow.

I sit on the rock beside me, and watch the colors.

Is this real? I ask myself. Is Dark Eyes real?

I am lost, lonely, and sad, but I need not feel this way anymore. I sit, watching the rainbow. "Why does he mean so much to me?"

In front of me is the dark figure of the Blue-Eyed Raven. "Your song—your heartbeat," he says. "Soon you will know the secret of why the bobcat smiles, and your loneliness will be gone."

"The spirit world is hard," I say.

"This is about physical, and all the choices," he says. "Be careful!"

"Granddaughter," I hear a familiar voice say.

Standing there by the tree is Grandfather Wolf in all his wolf power and all his beautiful, aged wisdom. His face is soft and wrinkled, his white hair pulled back in a pony tail; his eyes are dark and shimmery. His wolf cape is over his shoulder; his boots come to his knees and are etched in wolf skin.

"Grandfather, I'm sad. I'm very sad."

"Oh, why, Granddaughter? Why be sad? Listen to Big Music."

"I don't want to listen to Big Music. I don't want to be a part of the human race and I don't want to go back there with no answers."

"Granddaughter, you have the answers. Listen to the Blue-Eyed Raven—Change."

The wind circles us as he speaks.

"Watch the wind, like the smoke of a fire. It moves in circles and Changes. Nothing ever stays the same. To some it is death; to others it is life. Only lessons hold truths," he says, a softness in his voice.

I walk forward, a couple of steps past Grandfather, and there on the ground is a deer horn. I pick it up.

"The Black Horse will cross your path and together you will release the smoke. Perform the Ceremony of Forgiveness. Let go and understand we are human, and pain is the medicine of Proof. To know what Proof is, you must see your Dark Choice.

You must find the Blue-Eyed Raven and step through the Golden Door. It is the mind that holds the answers.

I hear the rattling of the bones calling me back.

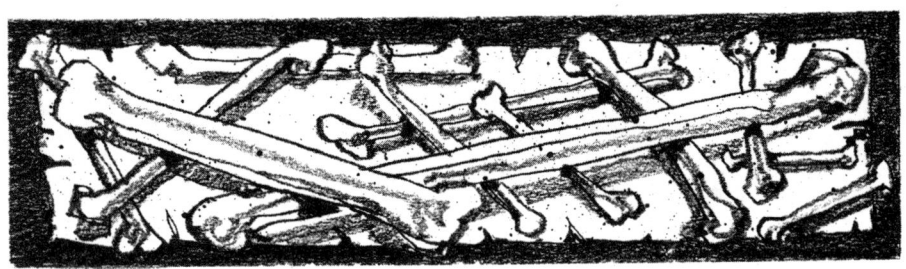

Teachings of Change—White-Tailed Deer Medicine

Change is one of my favorite teaching circles, because it excites me to know that no two minutes are ever the same, that no two days are ever the same, that no one person is ever the same. We might think of ourselves as the same, but because of Change medicine we are constantly moving upward, outward, inward, downward, backward, forward.

These are the sacred movements of life. When we utilize Change as a medicine, we draw it out and make a decision. Change starts when a Choice has been made. Choice has been made when the ceremony is complete, and the ceremony is complete at the end of Change, in the medicine Proof. That's what brings about Proof—the Choice. I would always hope that we apply Nurture before we do anything, and stay soft and gentle in our ways.

The energy of the deer makes Change quick. The movements within Change are four:

1. Different. You can see "different" in your gradual aging. However you see yourself today, you are different from what you were yesterday, and if you look 365 days ago, you can truly see the difference.

> *Example: Our physical existence shows life differences. One day you're sick and the next day you're well, one day you're sick and the next day you've passed on. Different can be seen in pregnancy. The pregnant person looks at herself one day and can't see any form changing, and the next day she sees the changing of form in the weight gain, and feels the discomfort of the physical structure of a life taking human form. The next day she looks up and it's time to deliver the child. But when she thinks about pregnancy, it's just a long blur of feelings brought about through Change.*

2. Give. Give is a positive movement clockwise or forward in life. It is the movement of stepping out around the medicine wheel. If your wheel is symbolically lying on the ground, you will step around the wheel and study each of the rocks as you move. Maybe you'll walk around the wheel three or four times before you realize that everything in life is the wheel, and you have been applying different parts of it from the minute you learned to remember that you could do it. Giving is a forward motion: It is never a taking motion, for then it would be to receive. I use an interesting symbol for "give." I draw a line and put an arrowhead at the top and an arrowhead at the bottom.

For giving, to me, is symbolized that way. It can also be symbolized as a circle, for there is never any give-away that there is not reception.

Many times in our lives we think we do things that we are never paid

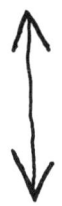

back for, like the tremendous amount of energy it takes to parent a child. We feel we never really get the appreciation or the reward that we deserve for being a parent. When we're honest with ourselves, each one of us feels that way, when in fact, we're not to receive anything for parenting, because parenting is an act of giving. What goes around comes around—giving is a circle. If you can see your opportunities and understand the great accomplishments of placing life on the earth, then you can truly understand parenting through the movement of giving energy or giving motion. Give brings about Change, in other words. You are not just stepping off in give, you have made a conscious Choice and you are now into the movement of Change.

3. Remodel. A physical Change that usually brings about a positive reaction, remodel can be an opportunity of Change, it can be a Choice of Change, it can be an actual finalization of Change. To remodel is to make better. Remodeling that makes worse is called a mistake. Remodeling happens by being organized. So when we are given our life, our physical existence, that is a movement of Change for the Creator. For the Creator is no longer alone when we have been brought into form. We are given an opportunity to do things and to bring about. There are simple things to remodel, like losing or gaining weight, changing your hair color or putting it back to normal, changing jobs—those are all forms of remodeling, and very much like Change, they happen gradually. When we Change our hair color, we don't just go snap and our hair color changes, we have to go about it in a process.

Remodel holds within it many words like thinking, organizing, prayer, rules, dedication, goals, work, and achievement. Therefore, remodel is a very powerful part of Change and is a physical action of Change itself for it brings about a difference, like from one hair color to another.

4. Transform. We see transform in our life as a newborn, an infant, a child, a teenager, a young adult, an adult, a middle-aged, a senior, an elder, and a relic. The steps of the life Change circle show us the transforming movements, the actual transformation of a human being. Transform is in the fourth position, for it is the step right before it is finalized and Change becomes Proof. Transform in the final stage of Change opens the doorway to Proof. The transform stages are part of Change, for they come right before birth.

Any time we have an idea and it doesn't work, we set out to find a different idea. We launch it, which is to give it away and to let it go. Then it moves around in the re-form stages, because it is not the same idea. It comes into transform when the new idea is actually born and established as a new thought. This is the cycle and the teachings of Change.

Aho.

Ceremony of the Cleansing of the Physical Body

The physical body consists of the mind, body, and spirit. In Rainbow Medicine teachings it consists of the mind, body, spirit, and emotions. When we cleanse our body a lot of people work on the physicality and forget the emotions and the spirit. In this cleansing ceremony, you are totally free to construct your own ceremonial setting. I suggest the ceremony be done early in the morning during the new moon, for that is a time when things are coming about. If you are trying to undo something in your body and cleanse it away, it is best to start the ceremony during the full moon and work the ceremony on out into the dark time of the moon.

Cleansing your body is a physical action, a mental action which is emotional, and a spiritual action. Spiritually, you can cleanse your body any time you know that your body needs to have a discharge or a release of a way of life, a teaching, or a fearful thought. For this ceremony, make sure you have your medicine blanket where it can go around your shoulders and keep you comfortable while you are moving through your cleansing.

The most important part of cleansing your body is remembering not to shock your system. Staying warm, staying safe, staying balanced in what is normal for you on a daily basis, is how you keep from shocking the system. I suggest physically that you drink plenty of fluids, that you have a low-fat diet, that you eat plenty of vegetables and fruit, that you have no alcohol, no drugs of any type, no carbonated drinks. Your sugar intake should be as low as possible.

When you are starting a Cleansing of the Body Ceremony, it is always good to seek out a counselor and a physician, a healer who understands your body, mind, and spirit, to help you balance yourself in the physical world, as well as following the ceremony from me or any shaman that you might choose. This healer specially needs to oversee any medication you might take for a physical imbalance that requires intervention through chemicals.

You'll need your journal and your pen, and I suggest you use a green candle, for you are making Changes in your life. You will also need your smudge bowl, fan, and herbs for the Ceremony of the Sacred Herbs, and any other things that you might need to perform your ceremony in an adequate way for you.

You are going to prepare a sacred place to do ceremony, and that means finding a quiet place where you won't be disturbed, where you can think. It should be a place you can come to when working on your cleansing process. In this ceremony, the actual cleansing can take up to two years. Some situations can take as long as five and some as long as eleven years. It is important to remember that when you just simply sit down to make a Change, it looks easy. But when you start working with it, you see that life is a web; life is the movement of the Medicine Wheel, and it crisscrosses itself. Everything is impacted by the smallest decision.

To start with, give yourself at least thirty minutes to an hour a day for the first one to two weeks of the ceremony. Then continue for three to seven weeks, working with yourself in the ceremony. Then go on over a longer period of time to make a Change.

Start by doing your Ceremony of the Sacred Herbs, and prepare to answer the following questions and organize yourself to make Changes.

Sit with your journal and light your green candle.

1. Who are you now? Who do you want to be? What is your physical shape, what is your hair color, how do you dress, what do you do for a job? Do you like the way you look, do you like what you do, do you like the way you dress, do you like yourself? Answer with the details of who you are in the physical life.

2. What are your sicknesses? List all or any of the illnesses that you might have. If you don't know or if you're concerned that you have a physical ailment or a mental condition that needs help, seek out the appropriate counselor, doctor, or teacher to work with you. List how you want to Change from these illnesses. Talk to a specialist. Organize and make differences by doing what you are told to do.

Example: *You have things about your face that you don't like and you want to Change them—Change the color of your eyes by wearing contact lenses, Change the shape of your face by having plastic surgery, Change your hair by dyeing it and changing the style.*

You need to go through the instructions and organize and understand what you are told by the specialists you'll be working with. When you are making decisions to work with the physical as you know it, it is important to understand that you can make any difference and come about with exactly what you need or wish to have in your life. Wholeness is achieved in physicality by settling with what you want. That comes about through having obtained the lesson of Obedience. When you make Changes in your physical condition, your illnesses, or anything in your life, you decide that it is going to happen and you make it happen.

3. What area in your life do you need to Change? Work through the problem by making a list of your likes and dislikes connected to the subject.

Example: *You want to do a total self-remake.*
(1) You don't like your weight.
(2) You don't like the way you talk.
(3) You don't like the friends you have.
(4) You don't like having chronic colds all the time.

You must sit with your self and understand why things happen.

(1) You pick your friends. You can make different Choices.

(2) You can Change your weight by working on it and becoming very healthy.

(3) You can take speech improvement classes, learn to Change the tones of your voice and how you present yourself through your words.

It is important for you to look very carefully at the areas in your life where you need to make Changes. By taking on the belief that you can Change anything, being organized, and carrying out what you need to have happen—you will make these Changes.

4. Journal how you are connected to your spirit while you are making physical Changes.

Example: One student, while going through Change, had family members hold his feathers and his Bible and burn a candle for him to achieve strength and safety while he was making Changes in his life. Others have had people do prayers for them, making prayer ties, keeping a light on for them, planting a plant and watching it grow in representation of their Changes.

List examples of your spiritual connection while making physical Changes.

5. What are your goals for physical wholeness?

Example: Wealth, good health, children, home, freedom, career, physical appearance, relationships. It is important to set out such goals as "It is my life, given to me by Great Spirit, and I have always wanted to be a healer." You then need to make out a list of the steps you will take to become one.

(1) Make my mind up that I wish to be a healer.
(2) Seek out classes, instructors, and instructions on how to become a healer.
(3) Find the type of healing I wish to do, make my Choice.
(4) Prepare financially.
(5) Study and become a healer.
(6) Practice.
(7) See the good in all the work, success, and job of organization that I have performed.

6. List your bad habits and how you want to Change them. Make lists of what it takes for you to Change a bad habit. Bad habits can be anything that makes you feel bad. They are not necessarily connected to physical actions.

Example: Some of your bad habits may be that you sleep too much, you think too much, or you worry too much.

Your habits affect your physical actions.

Example: You get angry quickly; therefore, you don't get anything done. You often hurt other people's feelings because of your anger.

7. Write a description of the new physical you, and show how you are connected to your spirit and how your spirit opens the door for you to live a good, solid, happy, physical existence.

> **Example:** *One student wrote, "I look healthy, I exercise, I quit all the sugar and sweet foods, and do prayers. I make out a list of what I do every day. I set goals for me to achieve my wanted physical existence. My goals are:*
>
> *(1) I accept myself, I image and see myself for what I am.*
> *(2) I set the goal to be healthy. I see a doctor, I study spiritual enlightenment and apply teachings of success to my life.*
> *(3) I surround myself with good people who have healthy lives, are clear spiritually and connected within their spirit and physical existence. They represent wholeness to me.*
> *(4) I do my prayer ties, say prayers, and have a close connection with my animal totems and spirit guides. I listen for circular communication with Great Spirit, knowing that everything I think and everything I choose, everything I might study, are the words of Great Spirit. I hold very strongly in my mind that I can make Changes and strengthen my connections any time I want.*
> *(5) I apply Choice medicine; I apply Ceremonial medicine; most of all, I believe in Change medicine—that I have the opportunity to make lists, see the things I don't like about myself physically, and seek out ideas and help from others, to obtain what I want.*

When you finish working with your lists, it will be important to look at your weaknesses and see if you need spiritual counseling, psychological counseling, or physical counseling, where you might need to seek out a bodyworker and obtain a better body through eating right and exercise.

You'll know from your goals and your conversation within the Cleansing Ceremony what you need to do to obtain your physical wholeness.

When you set out to make Changes in bad habits or do away with things that you don't wish to do, you must remember that you have to line out where you want to go. Making decisions and knowing the steps before you take them allows success within your new structure of physical existence. Don't rush, don't hurry, don't look at time.

Understand that you are going to give yourself two to five to eleven years to achieve physical existence goals. Going to school and getting an education doesn't happen overnight. Working hard and saving money doesn't happen overnight. Learning to dance, skate, jog, or work out at the gym properly doesn't happen overnight.

When you are working with your physical existence to bring about wholeness, I suggest that in this ceremony you simply accept yourself for what you are. Then you can see if it is possible to be what you really want to be. It may be that you are perfect, beautiful, wonderful, and enough, just the way you are. Ceremonially, it is important to continue to do prayers in green to allow yourself to understand that you are going through Changes. It is important to communicate with your family and friends within a Cleansing Ceremony, that you are going to lose weight, you are going to make habit Changes and continue to lose weight, or anything else that you set out to do.

Remember that Change brings about a new you. If you don't like that, you can always go back to who you were. But as you move along, I am sure you will find that when the time is up and you are the new you, you will have obtained your wholeness. Of course, by that time, you will probably have a new Change, or another Choice to make that will bring about a new Change, and you'll be off doing this Ceremony of Cleansing often throughout your whole physical existence.

Aho.

The Process of the Lesson of Action—Teachings of the Mule Deer

Action is movement. The mule deer is strong. It is stout and larger than the white-tailed deer. It is the spirit guide for the lesson of actions. It gives you the agility needed to move rapidly. Turning to the mule deer in spirit and asking for its guidance allows you to be strong and quick. Learning the lessons of action and performing action is the secret, I think, behind being a whole two-legged. Having physical wholeness by action is to Change your mind, accept quickly, forgive, and move on.

Your totem for the lesson of action stands quietly grazing on grass one minute, and running swiftly the next. It is important to remember, within the teachings of the process of the lesson of action, that you will have effect, that there will be a battle and there will be performance necessary for everything you do in your physical existence. This gives you the ability to complete the lesson of action and understand that physical existence is opportunity, it is adventure, it is school, it is learning.

The seven processes within the lesson of action are:

1. Perform. In learning the lesson of action, we see that our lives have gradual movement. We start out to mow the lawn, to wash the car, to go for a walk, to fix a meal. We go through the actions and this brings about the completion of the job or the project that we set out to do.

2. Undertaking. Most of the time we don't sit down and make out a list, unless it's a grocery list. In the old way, it is called thinking. In the new times, it is organizing—thinking about what we are going to do, making a list of things that we need to understand. The undertaking is the action that brings about success in anything we set out to do. By understanding, we have felt undertaking.

3. Energetic. To draw upon good health is a form of energetic action. To have good health is energy, boundless energy, that gives you the opportunity to achieve in anything you wish to do. Learning the lesson of action is to have the ability to be energetic. When we want to set out to raise children, take care of grandchildren, or obtain great intelligence within our physical existence, it takes an extreme amount of energy.

4. Battle. Within the lesson of action there is fight. There are many times in our lives where we don't want to make Changes. Changing a habit, getting a new job, going through a divorce, or getting married is a battle. It is a struggle within yourself—will I make it or will I not make it, how do I make it, what do I do to get it done? That's why growth and achievement start to emerge within the lesson of action—because the battle is there. You will either win or lose.

5. Moving. It is important to remember that you are not frozen. You can quit or start any time you want to. You can Change, move on, forget, dismiss, bring forth—all of these are movement. You have full control in your life to decide what you are going to do and what you are not.

6. Actual. The movement of actual within the process of the lesson of action is the spirit, the life, the universal connection, the all-ness that we share. We like to think of ourselves as unique and individual, but the actuality is that we are all human beings, male or female. We all sleep, we all eat, we all excrete, we all learn, we all forget. It is easy to separate ourselves from others, thinking that we are individual or unique. What uniqueness is, is simply the ability to sparkle. What individualism is, is the simple movement of taking responsibility. The actual within the action is acceptance, truth, common sense, and wisdom.

7. Effect. The final movement within the process of the lesson of action is when you have brought about, set up, and achieved your goal. Action happens when effect is seen, which simply means that cause and affect is the lesson of action. Something as simple as closing and opening your eyes affects. There is no way to break everything down and understand every tiny movement that it takes to achieve. Through the effects of your action, you see your goals, you see your dreams—a good relationship with your partner, a successful business opportunity, healthy and happy children, you feeling good about yourself and the Choices you've made. I feel that the strongest effect of the lesson of action is being happy. Holding onto that happiness as an actual physical wholeness is the most beautiful effect of action that a two-legged has the opportunity to feel.

Through the process of the lesson of action, remember you have the swiftness, the gentleness, the strength, and the large ears, like the mule deer. The ears allow you to find opportunities, or through prayer to connect with a new idea. Bringing about the lesson of action gives you opportunity.

Aho.

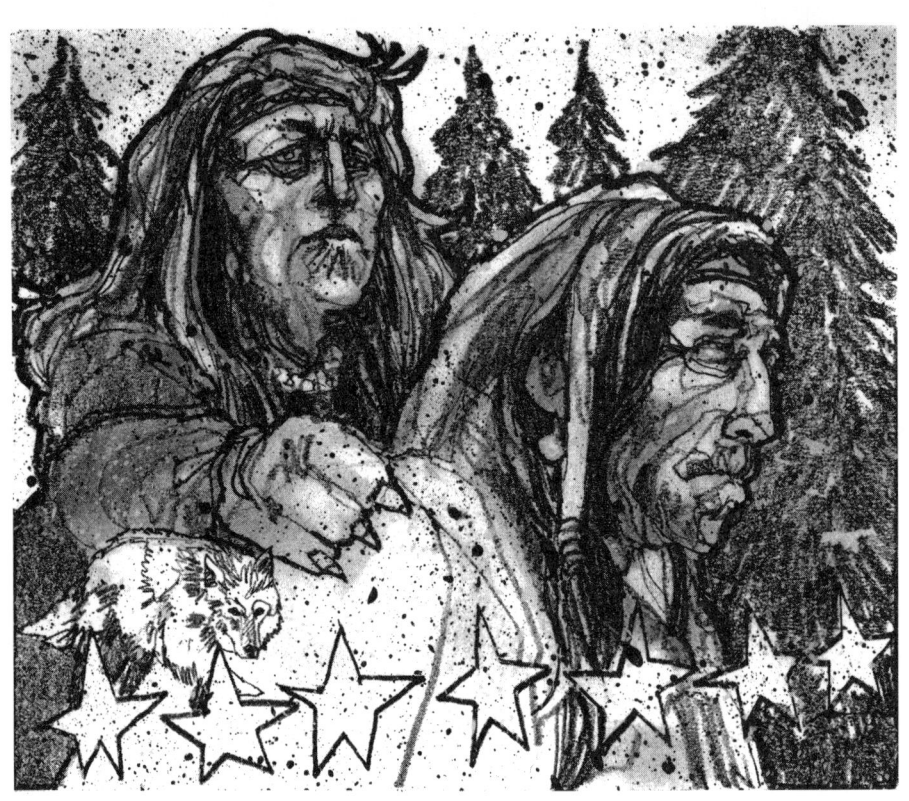

7
TALKING BONES—PROOF

Before me I see a path. As I walk along that path, the questions the students ask me echo in my mind. I think it is interesting that we reach a place in our lives where we begin to realize that we are all the same.

"Grandmother/Grandfather, why can't they see that? We all get married—or if we don't get married we wonder why we didn't get married. We all think we are unique. Each one of us thinks we are different from the next person, when if we look at the next person, we have about ten things alike. We are almost the same... Oh, well, it doesn't really matter, I guess."

I walk along, kicking stones. Beautiful stones—purple and white. They roll along in front of me.

"Snake Man, if you're listening, I sure wish you would appear, maybe around that next turn up there, and explain to me. Everyone lies. Everyone tells the truth. Everyone is the same, Snake Man. You're the same as Old Woman Rock, you're just different because you're a male, but you're the same. You've got your own problems, I bet."

I hear a swooshing sound around my head and the sky becomes a bright blue. The water is rushing past me, and I smell the smoke from a campfire nearby. It lingers in the air.

"People are not unique or different. They are individual in their personality. But alike as humans," Snake Man says, leaning against a tree. "Have you ever wondered if maybe there is no one else but you, and everyone around you is just a thought? Everyone else around you is just a dream, and you're the only one alive? You're the only one, and everything else is just your imagination—have you ever thought about that?" he asks with a grin—a devious grin, too—one that has mystery and excitement.

"Hmm, that would nice. That would be real nice, because I could just forget their problems. I could just think them well, and they would be."

"There you go, Wolf. That's what you do, and it will happen. I want you to see something."

He waves his hand and points. I see a wheelchair with a man with long hair, a braid. He is just sitting there. A woman comes and puts a blanket over him. Behind her I see a calendar—and I see a date. Then she rolls the man in the wheelchair onto the porch that looks out over the water, and he sits in the sunshine and nods off. I watch her come to him and try to wake him, but he is gone. The date on that calendar makes an impression that I will never forget. I look closer at the man, and I realize that he is Dark Eyes.

"No. No. Dark Eyes is not that way. He doesn't die. He stays alive forever, he—he can't get sick. He—he can't have these things happen to him, Snake Man!"

In spite of all the power I have received through the teachings of the totems and my experiences in Rainbow Medicine, I still don't understand death. I still don't understand pain and sorrow. I didn't think it was time for my mom to leave. I hardly even got to know my sister, and she's gone. I look at the people in the circle—the lady who thinks her marriage will go on for a long, long time, and her husband is so close to leaving; the young girl who tosses her hair in the air and has that excitement that comes from everything in life being new and the idea of a free life with no obligations.

They drift away. There is no one there. As I walk, I hear the hoot of an owl and the crunching of the leaves underneath my feet. I listen to the water rushing, feeling an emptiness inside.

I see a bright colored light—radiant color—surrounding a being standing in front of me. It is beautiful—a very dark blue. Between us there runs a fox, a silverish-blue fox. It runs into the woods, and weaving its way through the trees quickly, it disappears.

Getting closer to the being, I see an outstanding black horse, so black it is blue. As I come closer, the wildness of the horse becomes the freedom of a woman's hair. This woman's eyes are strong and intense. She is beautiful, small, muscular, physically fit, with a very comfortable feeling about her.

"What do you think, Wolf?" she asks in a soft voice. Her features are strong, her eyes wise. She wears a free-flowing blue denim skirt and a beautiful white blouse with tiny embroidered flowers; it is ironed perfectly.

"Who are you?" I ask.

She points to a necklace that she wears—with a black horse pendant and, on each side, two skeletons of little bones and black shiny beads. She has on black boots. In her hands she holds a black hat with an eagle feather attached to the hatband made of beautiful rainbow beads.

"Hmmph," she says. "I am the judge. I am the ultimate. Some call me Death. Some call me the Grim Reaper. Some speak of me as the Black Horse. Some fear me. Do you? Today I see the sadness. Today I know that you must not be really excited about my presence."

"Are you the one who makes the calendar date work?" I ask. "Are you the one who weakens his body and takes him away?"

"No," she says. "I am the one who gives him opportunity, as a graduation. I am the one who waves the wind so that he has the breath of life. You see, Wolf, those who are afraid of death do not understand opportunity. They have not understood the circle, the Medicine Wheel, the Sacred Hoop of Life. Death is not my name. They simply speak of me that way. Remember, Wolf, and you'll know me. Think for a minute and you'll see me."

I sit down on a rock. I am tired. I take a deep breath, and let it out. "I don't like what I see. It's the same thing I see in class. It's the same

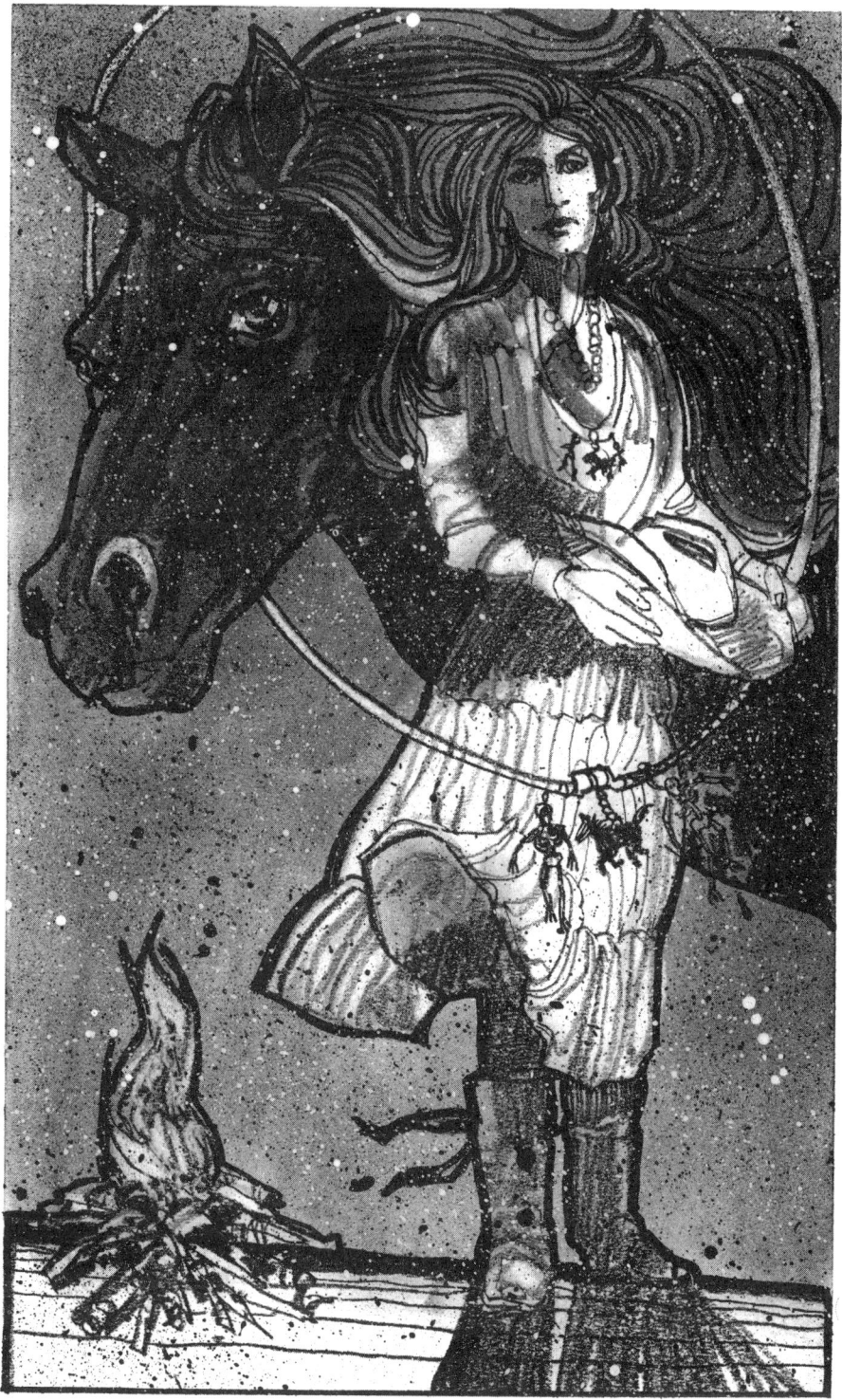

thing that everyone is afraid of. It's a constant worry of losing. It's constant loss."

"I don't think that's what Dark Eyes would want you to say," she smiles.

"Why does he die? How can a spirit die? Spirits don't die, do they?" I ask, tears in my eyes.

We talk and the river rolls past. She speaks of how we choose to die and I speak of how we do die. She speaks of how we choose to be sick, and I speak of how we do get sick. She speaks of how we want to be sad, and I speak of how we are sad. She speaks of how we have the Choice, and I speak of how no one does. She tell me that opportunity is what life is, and I tell her of lives of horror and pain and happiness that is fleeting. We talk long, long into the light of morning.

I build a fire and I listen. In the woods the little fox watches.

I love talking. Our words soar. We cover every topic that humankind has ever thought about, and then more beyond. I hear beautiful music all the time we are speaking. Every word is filled with notes of color and sparkling stars; sparks fly and my heart is filled with freedom.

"Wolf, remember this is all physical, and all comes to an end here," Black Horse says.

I hear a rattle, soft and slow. I look, and a bone person is standing there. It is joined by many little foxes.

Cold, still air is all around.

People rattle and move. They dance and dance on a circle, round and round. In the center of the circle is a house, small and cute, a little grass hut. I see a soft glow from the windows. The front door is open.

The dancers open the circle so I can come in. I start walking. I feel a soft rain as I enter the circle.

"You are in the circle of Proof now, Wolf," I hear a small voice say.

Faint blue lights swirl all around the house. Dark Eyes stands at the door.

"Come in. Welcome to my heart." He holds out his hand, and in it is a blue faceted stone heart. "Take my heart, it is a gift to you—a gift of Proof, that I am real and you will always be real to me."

I take the heart and go into the hut. "What a grand feeling in here," I say.

It is very cozy and warm, small but enough. It is only one room, built from grass and sticks, with a big log bed in the center. The bed is covered with a buffalo robe, and on the robe are red rose petals and a blue striped blanket. There is a stove with an easy burning fire and a coffee pot set on top. In the corner is a rocking chair. I look outside: rain is dripping off the porch, and I see the fox dancer prancing in the starry night.

Dark Eyes slips his arm around my neck. "I always wanted my own wolf," he says. "Stay with me, here, tonight."

"No," I say. "You are dying soon, and I don't want the pain."

"No pain—only Proof," he replies. "Proof is your medicine."

"No," I say. "There are too many others for you."

"Yes," he says, "and you are one of them."

"Spirits don't do this..."

"We are now physical, touch me," he says. He kisses me softly and I melt in his kiss.

"Why this?" I ask. "Spirit doesn't need this."

"Spirit is the kiss," he replies with warmth in his eyes. The light from the fire silhouettes our spirit as one on the wall.

"Look—it's us," he says. "We are us..."

"There is no us! I know this is only a dream!"

We drop to the bed where a night is a year. His deep voice embraces my heart. My eyes are interlocked with those dark eyes. Each kiss is long and full. I can feel his body deep within me. Warm and safe—I hold onto his heart. I can hear the rattles and smell the Fall night, the clean air. His soft skin next to mine is warm, our hearts beat hard.

I begin to cry.

"What's wrong?" he asks.

"I never want to leave," I say.

He smiles and brushes his wild hair from his face. "Leave? There is nowhere to go. I am your heart—you are my mind."

"Sex—spirits don't have sex," I said. "This is not real."

I go to move, and he pulls me back, wrapping his strong arms around me, rubbing his soft beard on my neck. Soft candlelight twinkles all over the room.

"Each candle is a prayer," he says.

I fall asleep, safe and warm, watching blue lights spin around my head.

The sun is in my eyes. I wake up by the rocks. The rainbow is gone. My Proof is my dream.

"He is my mind, only a dream."

"No, Proof is through the Golden Door," a strong voice says.

I look up. Across the way a black horse is eating grass.

"The way of the spirit is hard. No, the way of physical is hard. You belong to another, and through the Golden Door you will see," the wind speaks.

"Another? No, I have Proof." I hold out my hand, and in it is the blue heart.

I hear the rattling of the bones calling me back.

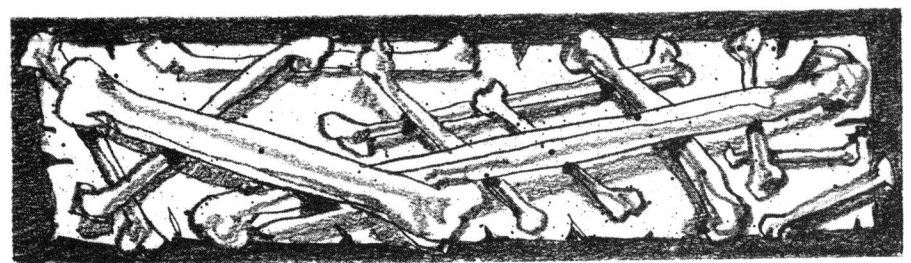

Teachings of Proof—Fox Medicine

I rely on Proof medicine a lot in my life. I was told a long time ago the old saying that the Proof is in the pudding. I asked my mom one time what that meant and she said, well, you put these things in the bowl and they end up being pudding. She said what they were, was milk, eggs, and other ingredients with their own bodily form, and when they came together, they made a new bodily form, which is Proof. Our human existence is spirit's Proof. Proof makes it very easy for me to see the four directions in the Medicine Wheel that are known as the Lesson Roads, the good and the bad, the right and the wrong.

I like to think of spirit as the center of those roads, and our physical existence the travel upon each of those roads. For in our existence, our humanness, we are free to have good and bad, right and wrong, and evil and godly. When you stand in the point of the center, you are a spiraling energy, a circle—outside your human form. When you take on form, matter, and existence, you have a being. Which is the Proof of all that is, everything that you can be or don't want to be, and that is our human existence. Each day we are given a test known as life. When we are a Fox Dancer, when we use fox medicine, which is Proof, we will be quick and clever. We will be masterful, graceful, and sparkling in everything we do.

You know, it's like the old saying, "He has a sparkle in his walk." That simply means that he is full of confidence, creative and powerful. As a Fox Dancer, he dances the sacred circle of life. In our human existence we see that circle, for when we are born, every baby is a sparkling energy. It is a brand new experience, a time for hope and opportunity. It is Springtime.

Then we move on into the Summer of our life and we are full of emotions and limits, because we are young. We are under constraint, because we are not adults. It is an intense time, for we are full of passion, but as young ones we are limited and told what to do. Often we become hot tempered and hot sexually.

We move on into our adulthood and we are ready. We are in the fullness of our life, the harvest time. We are looking death in the face for we know that age is upon us. From young adulthood all the way to full adulthood within the sacred circle of life, we are ready for everything that comes our way. Our maturity gives us the opportunity to work, to produce children and families, to become community members, and to bring forth our endurance as our mark, our legacy, our Proof of existence.

We step into the Winter of our lives when we become elders. We can be young elders; we can be in the young part of the Winter where it is still Fall but cool, and things are growing older and deeper.

We see the whimsical in our lives, we see the humor in it all. We see the different styles of clothing we have worn and the different ways we have painted our faces, worn our hair, and the different types of personalities we've personified. We understand when we are in the eldership of our lives.

It is important, in our Wintertime of our sacred circle, that we hold ourselves gracefully, that we move with the dignity and honor of the fox. For when we keep the twinkle and the sparkle in our eye as elders, we can then truly be remarked upon as a Grand parent. We can then truly be looked at as a Grand person. In the sacred circle of life we are a hoop—a spiral that shimmers and sparkles, that twinkles and glitters, that vibrates and resonates human existence.

Ceremony of the Breath of Life

TOOLS: *Cornmeal; sage; smudge bowl; fourteen colored ribbons four feet (1.2m) long—2 red, 2 orange, 2 yellow, 2 green, 2 blue, 2 purple, and 2 burgundy; a quiet place; medicine blanket; journal and pen.*

You can do this ceremony inside your home or outside. Inside, place your medicine blanket on the floor, smudge and bless yourself. Offer a prayer to Great Spirit. Be sure you will not be disturbed for at least 15 to 30 minutes.

Outside, find a quiet place. Make a circle of cornmeal large enough for your medicine blanket to be placed on the ground inside it. Step inside, smudge yourself. Be sure you are in a place where you will not be disturbed for 15 to 30 minutes.

1. Stand in the center of your medicine blanket and hold one of each colored ribbon in each hand. Start moving your arms around, allowing the ribbons to flow freely. The colors represent your physical body: red—your blood; orange—your energy; yellow—your muscles, cells and tissues; green—your bones; blue—your DNA coding and neurological system; purple—your brain; burgundy—your spirit.

Move the colored ribbons all around. Spiral them over you, down below you, in front of you and back of you. Watch the ribbons as they move uniquely, individually, and watch how they unite and work together. If you find yourself moving in a special rhythm, keep moving that way—for that is your physical rhythm. Enjoy watching the colors, let go of your worries and troubles, and be with your body.

2. Moving your arms up and down, back and forth, swirl the ribbon around your body and celebrate your physical existence. Think of your human self. Allow yourself to sit down and let the rhythm of the ribbons move around you. If you feel like lying down, do so. Move the ribbons all around and then let the ribbons become still. Feel the quietness of yourself. Think of all of you and appreciate your vehicle, your opportunity to experience wholeness and totality. Give a quiet prayer of gratitude for your human existence.

3. Stand and move your ribbons gently from side to side, in front of you and in back of you. With a gentle, peaceful sway, balance your body. Ask Grandmother/Grandfather to heal any sicknesses that you might

have and offer up gratitude for every minute of your physical existence. Feeling the ribbons swaying in the breeze, think of each day of your life as a gift from your spiritual grandparents that allows you to experience the test of life. Think of your physical experiences and give a prayer of gratitude for the lessons that you can learn. Let the ribbons gently hang down at the side of your body and understand that each color makes a total self.

4. When you are finished, step out of the circle and put away your sacred objects. Place the ribbons on your altar or in a sacred place where you can use them again, to breathe, pray, and be grateful for your physical two-legged existence.

Ceremonial Water Bowl

When you are performing sacred ceremonies it is important to have an altar. This can be a shelf or a spot on the floor where you lay a medicine cloth or medicine blanket and put your sacred objects on it. Your sacred objects are your "medicine," things that help you to live and grow, things that teach you and bring about understanding.

When we set our sacred altar and do sacred ceremony, we must always have objects representing the directions, such as a feather, dirt, a candle, and water. The air (East) is the feather. The earth (West) is the dirt. The fire (South) is the candle, and the water (North) represents itself.

There are many levels of spiritual teachings—many cultural differences—due to the timelines of physicality. I follow the vision of Rainbow Medicine in the way I present the four directions. As I understand it, spiritually, this sequence of the four directions was the first and will be the seventh way the directions affect the physical. You can find, in different teachers' instructions, the East governing water or fire, or the West governing water or fire—so remember that the four directions are often presented in different ways.

A sacred water bowl is a special bowl that you choose to hold water in. You can choose a clay bowl and paint your vision inside your bowl, or you can choose a special soup bowl that you eat from. The type of bowl doesn't matter, as long as it holds water and it is special to you. The more personal your bowl becomes, the more medicine it has, because it represents the water of life.

In each ceremony you perform, it is important to have a bowl that holds the elements within it. Your water bowl holds sacred water from the Earth Mother. It holds the shimmer and sparkle of the river and the brook. It holds the nurturing food of the lake. It holds the power and majestic movement of the ocean. It holds raindrops and tap water, and spring and creek tricklings. It holds the life force itself, the grand fluid of our existence—fresh water.

Gather your water from a sacred place, a place that brings you the power that is water. A water bowl is always empowered when it has water from the snow, water from the rain, from a lake, a brook, a creek, a river, and the ocean. I like to add cactus water—the fluid from the cactus that brings about life in an ancient way. I also like to put in a little apple and pear juice. I add many different fluids and liquids to my water bowl, so that I have a fluid representation of all the earth. It is important to use fluids that are pure and clean. Your water bowl should never be murky, yellow, mossy, slimy, or any color other than pristine, and perfectly clear.

Filling a water bowl and setting it on your altar is an empowerment. It is a representation of the life force of the Earth Mother. Always have a fresh water bowl present when you are performing ceremony. Remember that your water bowl speaks the lessons of the cloud people. It shares with you the turbulence and strength of the storm. Sit with your water bowl and listen to the waters of the Earth Mother. Listen to her fluids teach you of the blood of your body. Think of the fluids in your body and give yourself plenty of fresh water, for it is a healing force. When you are finished with your ceremony, pour the water on the ground so it can return to the Earth Mother.

Water from this bowl is the purest and most powerful medicine that you can put in your body, for we are fluid; we are the motion and the life force that Great Spirit has brought forth in its image.

Process of the Lesson of Solid—Crow Teachings

As we two-leggeds walk on this earth, we can be solid or we can be weak. In the Process of the Lesson of Solid, take out your pen and journal and write what you choose to be. Do you want to be weak, and if you do, write down why. Give all the reasons for why you would want to be weak.

Example: Someone can serve me, someone can worry about me, someone can use their life force taking care of me. I can be a burden to another. I can't do anything. I can't' achieve anything, and I am conscious of that, and I make it my choice to prey upon other people for my existence.

Then write in your journal what it would be like to be solid.
Example: I can, I will, I am. I am a person who has intelligence and knows how to use it. I have good study habits. I understand money is an exchange for time. I understand that family is a legacy and an honoring to my ancestors. I choose to be solid, for when I am, I have confidence, I am strong, I nurture myself, and I bring good to others' lives. When I am solid, I represent what I would want a child to be when it grows up. The things that I do, each one of them, have solid convictions behind them. I know that what I do shows other people the way in their lives.

These examples show you what I feel like when I am weak and when I am solid. Within the lesson of solid, now do the same. Bring forth your feelings of what you are when you are solid.

In the Lesson of solid it is important to learn the following seven words:

stable	**fine**
good	**complete**
financially sound	**sturdy**
excellent	

I recommend that you discuss this with an elder. Elders are not always aged. The definition of an elder, spiritually, is one who knows, one who is right, one who brings about good in his or her walk of life. Physically, an elder is someone who has white hair, and that means from the beginning when the first few white hairs start. The elder has stopped her menstrual cycle, or is one who is strong and capable of providing for his or her family, and is respected in the community for goodness and honor. Often, people become elders when a family member dies, and they have to take on the responsibility of being the oldest in the family. The type of elder I wish you to connect with is a teaching elder, one who knows what he or she is talking about, one who has experience, one who does things with respect. Your elder should show principles and virtues, be moral and honor the Sacred Circle of Marriage. He or she should bring honor to those he or she walks with, and live the good Red Road. If no elder is available to you, you may also do a shamanic journey and speak to Old Woman Rock or Snake Man.

When you are talking to your elder, ask yourself the following four questions for each one of the seven words above.

1. What is _____?
2. How do I apply that word to my life?
3. Can you show me examples of how to be_____?
4. What will I gain in my life by being this _____?

To achieve the process of the lesson of Solid, you need to study those seven words and bring them into your life. You can use me as one of your elders, if you want, in the lesson of Solid. To learn the lesson of Solid it is a good idea to have at least four different teachers' opinions for each word.

Stable. I see "stable" as someone who knows that human existence is a test—that you are tested on whether or not you do good versus bad, know the difference between right versus wrong, and are able to reflect godly versus evil. I believe that stable is achieved when you are healthy mentally.

Good. I believe that you learn the lesson of Solid when you know what good is—that good grows, that it produces, that it brings forth. I see good as education, as art, and creativity. I see it as a skill, as a trade. I see it as parenting, as truthful, honest, and respectable.

Financially sound. I believe that to be Solid you have to understand that a dollar is a dollar and that an hour is an hour. You have to know the value of a dollar and know the value of an hour. You also have to understand that an hour is time in your life and a dollar is a measure of money, which is a bartering tool. I think that "financially sound" most often is misunderstood: that we should look at ourselves and see that we are capable. If we are capable, then we are financially sound. We need to be alert to our surroundings, keeping up daily with the world around us, because those two pieces of the puzzle give us the opportunity to call upon our spirit, to look within our vision, to ask our elders—and from that anything can be learned. To become financially sound you have to know who you are, what your vision is, where you want to go with your life, and what you want to offer your children. Financially sound is not what size house you own, or how many homes or boats you have, or if you are able to have a vacation and pay for it. It isn't even that you have a job. To achieve financial soundness takes discipline, organization, commitment, and hard work.

Excellent. I see excellence as the ability to set your goals and to achieve them. Achievement is excellence, to me.

Fine is defined in my lifestyle as acceptable. When things are fine, you can live with them. No one said you have to live in a seven bedroom home. A one bedroom cabin, a one bedroom trailer, one room, one car—anything is fine as long as you are happy with it. I like to define fine as happy. I like to define happy as being in line with your purpose or intention.

Complete. To be Solid cannot be achieved without completeness. Many people think they cannot be complete if they are not married. To be complete, you have to know what you are and what you need. Sometimes your job requires you to be unmarried, but you go ahead and get married and then can never achieve the full potential of your job. Complete is having the ability to ask yourself where you will be in twenty years and who can be there with you. It's the intelligence and the wherewithal to look at your hobbies, at your needs and wants, at your vision, and know what it will take to achieve those things. Often when we think we need children, family, half-sides, and marriage partners, it is simply a whim that we have due to abandonment and loneliness. So we marry, we have children, or we stay in the same community—close to our friends and family—and we become restricted and limited: We never complete our own walk on the Red Road and achieve our purpose.

Sturdy. Sturdiness comes from your inner core. Inner core is experience. So how you were parented is very important in your sturdiness. I think a tree could raise a child, if the child could look at the tree and live like a tree. That's a strong example of what sturdy means. I believe that the child would recognize that it's not a tree, and would die, because we all know that an infant wouldn't know how to get milk from a tree.

So our parents play an incredibly important role in our first years of life. We are able to depend on them and not be lied to, given racial insults, abandoned, or raped.

We need to look at our parents and see the Rainbow Medicine Wheel. For me to be sturdy I must have confidence in my spirit. I must be strong in my emotions, and I must nurture my body and have color in my mind always. Then I will sing the sacred song of Great Spirit, for then I will know the sun and the stars and the moon. I will respect the earth and will drink of the water and warm myself by the fire. These are my ways which I pass to you. They have worked for me, and they are what my mom taught me to do.

The crow represents the number fourteen. The crow is a symbol of the judge—the Judge of life and death. The crow gives us the opportunity to look at our boundaries. I personally think that to achieve solidity, we must have boundaries. When you are taking that walk outside and you hear the crow call, look at it and think about the number fourteen. Understand that when you start with the number one, you have a long way to fourteen. But when you reach fourteen, you are at the end. That is death. That is why I teach that the crow represents death and the call of the shaman.

To finish your homework with the lesson of Solid, go forth and experience four different elders' teachings about the word Solid and then come up with your own statement of whether or not you are weak or strong. When you have achieved that, you will have identified a large facet of your personality. Don't get caught up on the Blue Road and bury your head in the sand, filling your heart with material pleasures, or get angry with those who try to guide and direct you. Open your heart to true spirit. Set boundaries, set goals, set disciplines, and achieve—for that will be Solid and you will have learned the Process of the Lesson of Solid.

Aho.

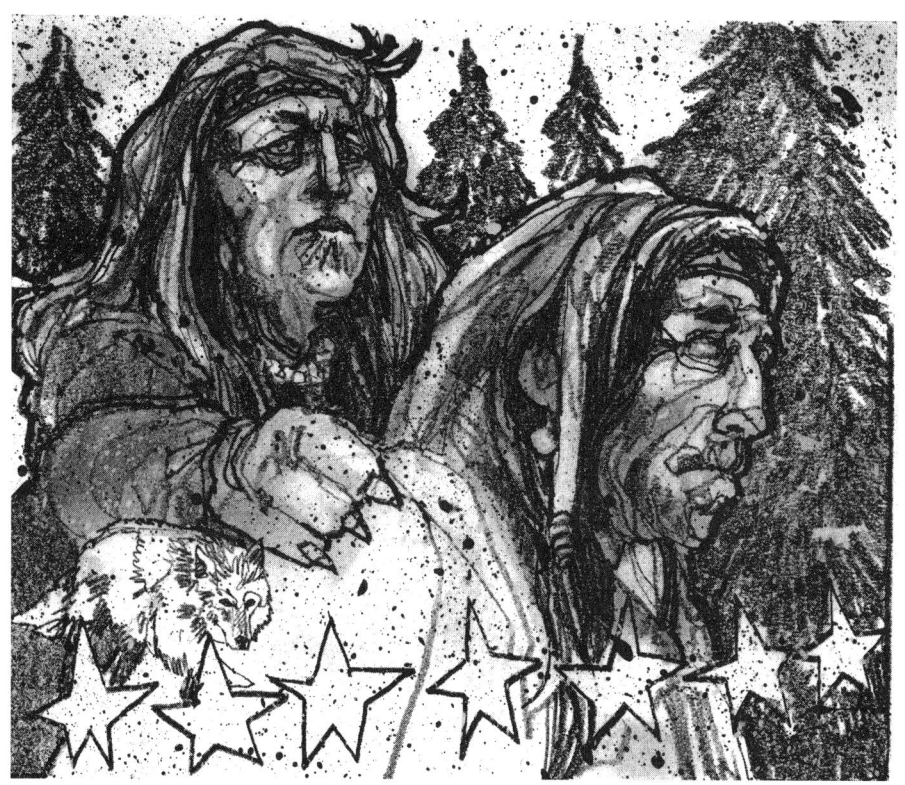

8

THE SONG OF THE BONES— TEACHINGS OF REAL

I breathe in and out, and relax. It is quiet and peaceful. I walk around the Medicine Wheel quietly, watching the prayer candles twinkle in the night. I think of what one student said tonight, and I find great joy in her words. "I think I understand what you're saying, Wolf," she said. "We are each a piece of God. Maybe I don't say Great Spirit, because I'm not Native American, but if I understand right, the Medicine Wheel doesn't have racial eyes. In other words, I think that there is a difference between physicality and spirituality, but they're the same as the words Real and reality. Right?"

I looked at her and said, "Exactly," and I saw the light go on in her eyes. I knew that she understood something that mattered to her. As I stand on the stone of Real, I know that spirituality is about that. Each one of us figures out for ourselves what we believe. Her example of Real and reality is exactly the truth. I bend down and blow out the last spirit candle. It is dark in the Medicine Wheel and I am standing close to the North gate. These seven people are very special, I think. Matter of fact, anytime people understand a small fraction of why they exist, I think they are very special.

I breathe in and out, and I hear the leaves rustling around me as the late Fall wind kisses each limb of the tree. It's been a pleasure to watch these students experience their physicality and see that physicality is spiritual—that everything we do is spiritual, because we are all made in the image of Great Spirit. It is interesting to remember the student who realized that if you were to murder, you would be saying that God murders. Or if you were a sexual predator, you would be saying that Great Spirit is a sexual predator. Often we want to separate our actions from the Creator and say no, I'm this way and God's that way. If we follow the teachings of Great Spirit, it is very clear that we are all Great Spirit. I can't countenance murder and sexual abuse as the purity and perfection of Great Spirit. But what I do know them to be is behavior brought about by mental illness.

I like what one student said tonight, "Monkey see, monkey do." That old cliché is true. Humans see monkeys perform in ways that we think we should mimic.

I walk to the East gate and turn and look back into the medicine wheel. It is a beautiful sight whether the candles are on or off, whether sunlight shines on the circle or moonlight, or whether the shadows of darkness are the stones of lessons. The medicine wheel holds within it the truths.

I hear a clicking and clanking above me. I look up and there are some old chicken bones, a few turkey bones, and a couple of bones that I assume are cattle bones, along with some forks and spoons tied to some sticks. They are hanging in the tree by the Medicine Wheel. The wind blows them and they clink, clank, and tinkle softly. I start to walk away from the wheel thinking how privileged I am to have the honor to provide a place for a student to have a tree of Real. The Medicine Wheel holds within it teachings of Real.

I decide to sit by the tree and listen to the sounds. I lean against the tree and listen to the tapping and clanking of the objects clicking together in the wind.

Before me I see him standing.

"Why do you have a tear in your eye?" he asks.

"It's hard to come up with the words, Dark Eyes. But the section of physicality in the Rainbow Medicine Wheel, the voice of the sun and the moon and the seven stars has overwhelmed me. I've seen you grow old and it's scary to me. Because death is a Real thing on the Earth Mother. I felt that in my mother and the passing of my sister. I've known death before, when I've lost animals," I say. "But the thought of you dying scares me."

He walks over, places a blanket around my shoulders, and says, "Come with me, I want to show you something."

We start to walk along a path through the trees. We come to a clearing and in sunrise we stand, looking out at the purples, the pinks, and the oranges. We look at the view of the mountains and the fog that lies as quietly as the holy smoke that comes from the sacred pipe.

"You don't know who I am, do you, Wolf?

I shake my head. "No, since I walked into my vision I can only have faith. When I first saw you dance across the river, I knew I needed to follow you. Remember I told you, you are my mind and I am your heart. I have given you my heart."

Standing behind me, he wraps his arms around me and holds on tight. "I gave you physical touch. I gave you my physical presence, so you would always remember who I am and that you would not die. It is important that you have a warm heart, and that you know that we are one. For, as my mind you are my thoughts, and that is Real medicine to me. I think on the Earth Mother they call it love. It is at the core of blood and family. It is at the core of friendship, honor, and respect."

We stand and watch the sun rise and reflect on the red rock in the mountains. The snow has come early this year and etchings of snow embrace the mountain sides. I don't want to leave his embrace and move away, because I'm afraid that he will disappear. I turn slowly and look him in the eye.

"When we danced on the river, I was a child. I'm not a child anymore. It's been a long time. When you go around the wheel and you come to this spot, you're an adult," I say to him.

"Wolf, in the spirit world, you are a spirit. You can be anything you want to be. Look." He put his hand on my shoulder and changed into a young man. "I'm only twelve," he says with a squeaky voice, and then he changes back into the form I know.

"Wow, that was fun."

"Yes, it is fun here," and he changes into a beautiful stallion in front of me, then an elk, then a cougar, and then an enormous, beautiful cottonwood tree. Then he is himself again. "Try it. Be anything you want."

I become a chocolate cake; then I am a stone of radiant beauty. Then I become a wise person—someone whose opinions I've always wanted to know. I stand there and think their thoughts. Then I become a feather and float in the wind. Then I am myself, looking at him.

He says, "Give me your hands."

I give him my hands. I place first one in his, then the other. He begins to spin us around. We spin around and around and around. We put our feet toe-to-toe, and go round and round. We became one spinning force. He raises our hands high in the air, and we become one—a spinning source of turquoise blue light. The light gets deeper, darker, and richer, until it is a dark purple. Then we stand still and I look in his eyes. He puts his hand on the side of my face and says, "You must let go. *You must let go, so that we are together. We are the same, one mind and one heart.*"

My blanket is wrapped around us tight—from the spinning—and I stand pressed against him, listening to his heart beat.

"Breathe your breath of life from my beating heart." His gentle hand caresses the side of my face and the warmth of his life becomes my spirit. "When you go to the earth you will walk with one. You will know him as the Blue-Eyed Raven, you will know him as yours. You will walk with him as his half-side and you will stand in your wholeness with him. But I will know your curiosity," and he begins to grin. There is a devilish, childlike look in his face that touches my heart and makes me soar.

"Things are not always the way you think they are. Things are the way they are to be. You must listen to the Song of the Bones, for you are a human now and I am your heart. You remember now, and it is a long ways away from where you are. For in a moment you will look straight ahead and there will be the clinking and clattering, clanging, and tinkling sounds that you drifted here to me with," he says. "It doesn't matter what you do or where you go, for you are walking your earth walk, and when you are here, there is nowhere to walk. There is nowhere to leave or to go, for we are the spirit walk."

I feel the tears welling up in my eyes, for I know soon I will let go of his hands, and there is nothing more empty than not to be able to feel his soft skin, not to be able to look into the eyes of wisdom that can tell me stories and explain why. "I will have to let go soon, and I know that."

"No, that's like how I allowed you to embrace me physically. On earth, evidently it is a compliment to become physical with another person, and only now you'll feel this emptiness, for you are in Real. When a human being is in its two-legged form, it lives with both halves of realness. When we are human, we are Real and we are in reality. That is where you are now. I will take you soon to a place that they speak of—the elders, the ancestors—called the Golden Door. When you go in the Golden Door, your human knowing is complete. Now you must walk in the Lesson of Full. Can you let go of me and know that I am you?"

I take a deep breath and tremble inside. I remember her—her hands slipping over his shoulder, her coldness, her intensity, as she ripped us apart. It felt as if the fibers in my body were tearing my heart out of my body.

"But if I let go of your hands, she will come, the Deer Woman. She will take you. I have seen this and I have seen the date on the wall and I know that you will die."

He is bare-chested and around his neck hangs a bag made of elk skin. It has a flap that closes with a turquoise button. He opens that bag and takes out a sparkling blue powder. It glitters and glistens. You can hear twinkling sounds all around it. He throws it up over my head. "Forget that. Your fears are balanced, and you are home at the river. Know that the mother river balances you, and when you stand there in her beauty, the Song is what you have. The movement of the sacred spiral strengthens your heart, and you remember the purpose of your earth walk. You and I," he looks deep into my eyes. "Let your head drop and your eyes close."

I did.

"Quietly breathe," he says. "Take a soft gentle breath and, as you do, smell the powder that I have sprinkled on you, and listen to the Song of the Bones."

I begin to breathe the wonderful aromas of Spring days, the smell of the ocean, the scent of leaves burning in the Fall, of fresh mowed grass, of honeysuckle and hyacinth, jasmine, and gardenias. I smell freshly washed towels and babies, and cotton candy. I hear children laughing, old ones singing, flutes and drums. The air caresses my hair and touches my cheeks.

I open my eyes and there beside the tree in front of me stands a girl, a young one, in her teens. Her hair is long and black, with white streaks in it. She has a black cloth wrapped around her from the waist down. Her top is covered with a cape made from skunk skin and deer hide. She wears one necklace of nuts, rocks, and the claws of a skunk, and another with seven keys on it.

"Hello," she says. Her eyes are black with shiny silver stars in the center. Her nose is slightly pointed. Her features are long and narrow. She is thin, very spirited and energetic, full of zest and zeal, and focused. "I'm glad you're here. I'm glad you've come to the Tree of Real. Are you enjoying the Song of the Bones?"

I listen to the clinking, the clattering, the jingling, and jangling of the silverware tied on the sticks in the tree. "I can hear it, yes. Who are you?"

"I am the lesson-bearer of Full. I have come to ask you if you have had enough. I want to know if you have hurt yourself enough and if you're ready to live, or if you want to continue to believe that people can destroy you. My job is to tell you what is right and to show you that you are Complete. It is mine to share with you the news that no one can hurt you but you."

Her voice is soft and she is straight to the point. When she speaks I can hear the song of the rattle that hangs above her. Each bone makes its own hollow sound.

"What clan are you from, or what spirit are you?"

She smiles and says, "I am Shenonna. Shenonna is s-s-s-s-skunk medicine. I am Shenonna Woman."

"Is Shenonna skunk?" I ask.

"No, my name is Shenonna. I am skunk medicine. I am Skunk Woman, Shenonna Woman, that's me."

I say, "Aren't you a child though?"

"Yes, I am a young woman. I am here at the Tree of Real to understand that I must carry skunk medicine. There will be those who think less of me because I do not have a Grand medicine like eagle or elk or

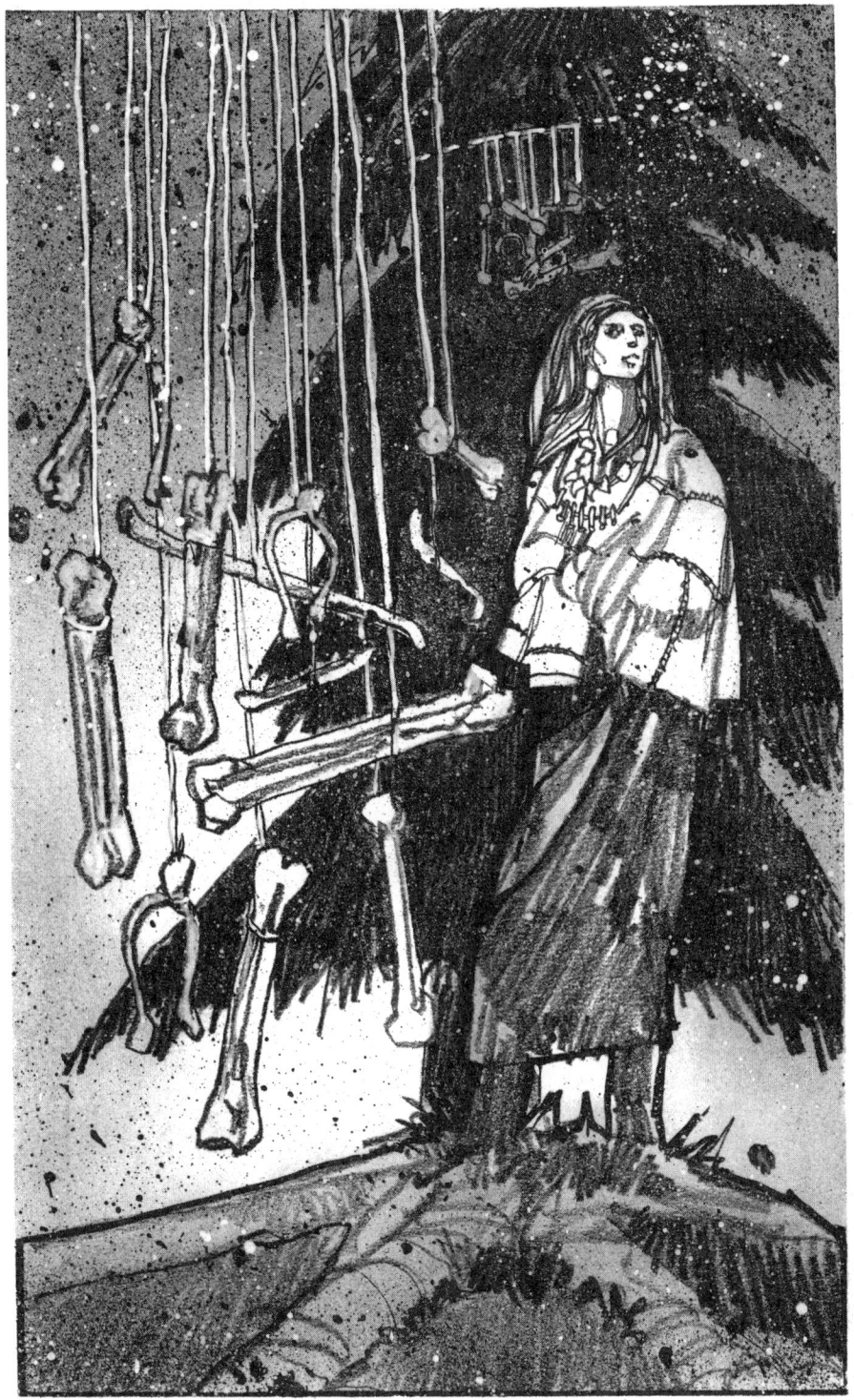

bobcat or lynx. I am skunk medicine, Shenonna Woman. Your lesson of Full calls you to complete your walk in the Rainbow Medicine Wheel section of the physical existence. You go and teach the answers of why people live as two-leggeds."

She smiles and taps the chimes above her head. When she does, the whole tree begins to sing with sounds. I hear deep clinking, tiny jingling, clattering, clicking—large sounds, rich and full. The sounds of the tree overcome me and I find myself falling backwards. I feel as if I am rolling down a hill. I go a long ways down. Then I feel myself stop. Cool, rushing water is all around me. I have rolled into the river and I am lying in a shallow pool of cool water, staring up at the bright Grandmother Moon, whose full face is smiling at me. As I look at Grandmother, I begin to realize what Full is.

"Yes, Granddaughter, I am Grandmother Moon," and her silver silhouette passes me with the familiar scent of river flock, the native flower of this river. Its smell is sweet and tender, that of jasmine. It touches me with memories—memories of days I spent at home, of a time of fulfillment, a time of peace.

I hear familiar laughing—Grandmother/Grandfather Wolf, my mother and sisters, friends that I have grown with on the earth plane, students whose laughter I love. My heart is filled with joy.

"Grandmother Moon, I am full."

She laughs and says, "Yes, Granddaughter. I am Grandmother, and you are Full. Listen, Granddaughter," and I listen to the song of Big Music, the birth of souls. "This is the Song of Creation, the Song of the Bones."

It is a sound of angelic voices, women's voices, singing—sounding so beautiful it takes my breath away and leaves pictures of the mountains etched in my mind. The beauty fills my soul.

I hear the rattling of the bones calling me back.

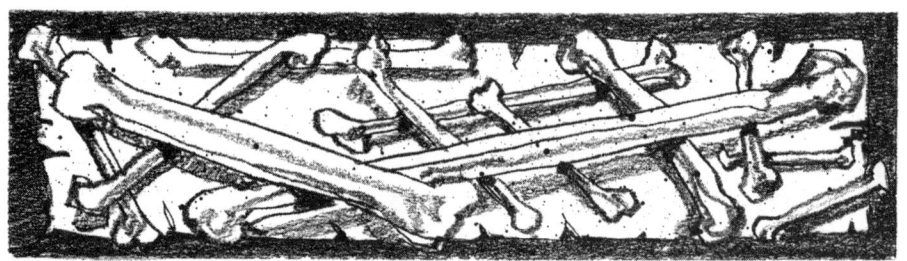

The Teachings of Real—Skunk Medicine

There are many times in our lives when we think we're doing something that is Real. What we set out to do is what we think we should do, and we do it because it opens doors, or it takes us away from pain and abuse. It moves us outside where we can be in the fresh air and feel the Earth Mother touch our heart. Sometimes when we think we are Real, we do what we do for attention. Sometimes what is Real to us is an illusion, and we're in the wrong place at the wrong time. Sometimes we feel that in another time or another place we could do whatever it is—sing the song and be professional, be the model, own the business, have enough money, earn the acceptance of all the people, be the star.

But what is Real is who you are. What is Real is what you can do. What is Real is the outcome of how you apply yourself. In Real medicine, you are given a medicine that allows you to accept, focus, and bring about who you really are. It allows you to *be* who you really are. Often in life I see people want to be something they are not, want to have things that they don't need, want to go places where they don't need to go. Because of that, we have many choices and lots of waste on Earth Mother today. Because they don't know their realness, they think that it is who they love, who loves them, how much they have, or how they look that makes them successful and happy. When truly, in human existence, Real is right, it is whole, and Real words are hard.

When we set out to achieve a goal there are avenues of success that go along with the goal that can sometimes be quite costly, because they are not related to the Real you.

It is easy in our existence as humans to put on airs and try to be what other people want us to be. It's hard to turn and tell the truth. Real medicine teaches us that sometimes we have to say things to people that hurt their feelings. We have to point out truths to people, which will set them in ways that open opportunities to them, where they can be successful.

Sometimes realness comes for us in such a way that we have to accept that we stink. When we think of a skunk we always think of its smell, and we look on it as a bad thing. Where did we learn that? The smell of the skunk is its sharpest claw—that means that the skunk has the ability to protect itself with a pungent odor.

Over the many years I have been doing work connected to mental health, one of the things I have noticed is that when people don't feel good, they don't smell good. When people are depressed, severely alcoholic, or addicted to drugs, they lose touch with their vanity. They lose touch with the desire to wear fragrant oils and perfumes, to represent the smells of heaven, to walk as a spirit and represent the spirit world with their aroma.

Realness comes to us in very pure ways. Poverty and abuse don't smell good. Those who are depressed and chemically dependent don't celebrate pleasant fragrances. I like to think of the rotting flesh, the foul smells of life, as an absence of Real. Though evil does smell awful.

We'll put our hand up in life and say, "I'm no skunk. I don't need to be told I stink." When our behavior, our choices, and our intentions stink, sometimes we don't want to hear that. Sometimes we don't want to say that to someone. But that's how it is. In Real medicine, your realness opens doors for you to stand in your Grandness, to look at the reason and smell the reason. Sometimes when we think it is over, it has just begun.

Aho.

Ceremony of the Tree of Real

TOOLS: *A piece of butcher paper four feet (1.2m) square, or a poster board (large); finger paints—red, orange, yellow, green, blue, purple, and burgundy; newspapers—enough to lay down a 5' x 5' (1.5m square); a towel that you can wipe finger paints on; sage, matches, and smudge bowl; a place where you won't be disturbed; a journal and pen.*

1. Go to the place where you have decided to do the ceremony of Real. Light your sage, place it in your smudge bowl, and fan it with your hand or a feather, cleansing and clearing the energy. After you have smudged the area, lay down a 5' x 5' square area of newspaper. Then place the butcher paper or poster board on top of the newspaper.

2. Open your paint jars and mix them up. Place the colors in front of you and close your eyes. Reach out and select your color. You can choose one or several. With your fingers, put the paint on the bottoms of both feet. Stand up and place one foot at a time on the poster board or butcher paper with your eyes open. Walk on the paper any way you wish to, or stand. After you have made your footprints, step off and clean the paint off your feet.

3. Close your eyes, mix up the paint jars, and select the paint you wish to use next, to paint your hands. You can use one or several. Choose the paint, and with your fingers, color the palms of your hands, or just one hand. Place your handprints on the paper in all different ways.

4. When you finish placing your handprints on the paper, clean off your hands and close up your paints. Take out your journal and set a topic, or an intention, for the painting that you have done. Set your intention on the Real aspects in your life—buying a car, for example, or having a happy marriage—for your painting represents the Real aspects of a question or a situation that you are dealing with. In the back of this book, you can look in the Colors section and see the medicine and lesson words for all the colors in the Rainbow Medicine Wheel.

Your footprints represent the lessons that you are learning or need to learn about the topic. Apply the words that go with the colors you selected for your footprints.

The colors that you have applied to your handprints are the medicine words that you need to apply to the situation to make it work the way you want it to.

> ***Example:*** *You have placed many red footprints on the paper. This means that you need to learn, and are learning, all of the red lesson words. If you have used different colors, follow the lesson words for the different colors. If you have drawn pictures—not just handprints or footprints—you are organizing and working hard to understand and apply your lessons to your life. If you have only used your fingers or toes, then you are just beginning to learn the lessons.*

5. When you are finished with your paintings, you can place them on the floor around your altar area, hang them on the wall, or title them and keep them with the intention or question that you have asked, making a portfolio of readings that you have presented to yourself from the Tree of Real.

6. When you are finished with the ceremony, put away all the tools that you have used, wash out the paint from the towel, and put away your ceremonial paper appropriately.

7. Take your smudge bowl and smudge the area, offering thanks to Great Spirit for the lessons you are learning.

Process of the Lesson of Full—Ant Teachings

When I achieved my lesson of full was when I understood what ant teachings are. I can say that full is one of the harder lessons. The process of the lesson of full was taught to me by a great warrior. I was striking out in my young years at my child abuse and issues that are connected to being a mixed blood Caucasian and Native American. I carried a lot of anger around with me and I wanted to take it out on education, and say the schoolteachers were the wrong ones. I wanted to take it out on religion and say the church was the one at fault. I wanted to follow a hollow and brutally vicious philosophy and believe that maybe a devil caused my abuse. Then I realized an ant's life tells the absolute story of complete and whole. An ant shows us that we need nothing but ourselves. We are designed to survive and to survive we need food and we need to reproduce.

I can't say that I would want to be an ant. I feel that human existence is a wonderful test and that that test is an opportunity to experience our feelings. But ant medicine has shown me that when times are rough I can let go. The lesson of full itself is being complete with one's wholeness.

Wholeness is being intact, with an understanding that you are physical and spiritual. Wholeness is a spiritual blessing to our physicality. Wholeness is physicality, and the only thing that can disrupt our wholeness is our mental health.

In our wholeness, we reach a point of full, and fullness turns into a learned lesson when we accept the idea that our physicality is our dark side.

I like to think of our physical emotions as reactions. This gives us the opportunity to apply Choice or to make Changes by drawing on our spiritual teachings—which means simply applying our medicine. Our human emotions change quickly. Sometimes you can call them fleeting feelings. When we walk with an understanding of our wholeness, we have strong orange medicine working for us, because we are balanced.

It is important to remember that our wholeness is brought about by understanding the four directions within us. Within those four directions, all things are possible.

When you understand that nothing can hurt you, then you can give your power to the one sacred movement—knowledge.

When you reach a point of enough in your life, you put your foot down and say to yourself, "I will follow the sacredness and I will honor the morning. I will give thanks at noon. I will be grateful in the evening, and I will go to sleep in complete understanding that this is the day that Great Spirit has given me—and it is not a dress rehearsal." When you apply these four movements—giving thanks, being grateful, being able to sleep, and noticing the sacredness in your life—the lesson of full is complete.

The ants spend all their time finding and retrieving food to share with each other. The next time you want to feel the experience of full, take a bread crumb—something that you might take for granted—place it in an ant bed, and watch the ants work very carefully on the bread crumb. Reflect back that this bread crumb means nothing to us—it is something that we might sweep up and throw away, but for them it is food. After they consume something we take for granted, they are content and able to survive another day. It is the same if we give them a piece of our skin or a strand of our hair—for we lose those things every day and either take it for granted or don't even notice. Watch the ants celebrate survival.

Sit with your journal and make a list of the things in your own life that are the lesson of full—or where you see the lesson of full.

Aho.

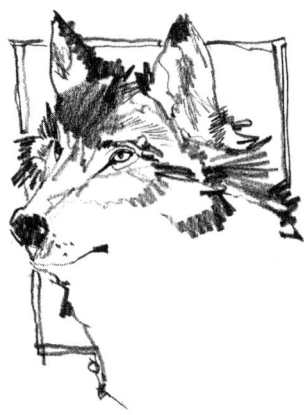

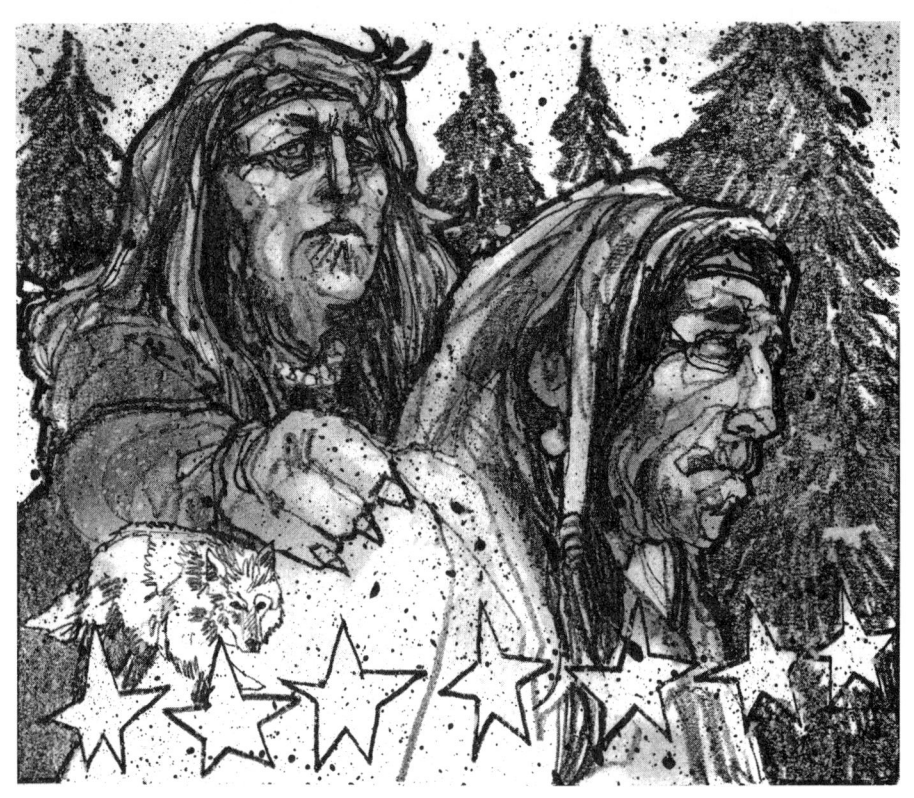

9
THE GOLDEN DOOR— GRAND

I breathe in and out, and I continue breathing. I watch a group of students bow their heads in prayer as they decide whether they want to go on. I see two standing at the gate who are new, who will come to this group. They studied long ago and they want to come back and go on to the North. They wait patiently, as the others make up their minds.

I ask, "Who here thinks the teachings of Rainbow Medicine are Grand?" and six of them hold up their hands. The two new ones at the door raise their hands, and there are eight of them.

So it's on to Wolf Medicine. My mind drifts and listens to the memories and to the story of the vision. Quiet comes to the Talking Circle; there are no students and the fire is dying out.

Each ember glistens and burns. I see a path in the fire and Old Woman Rock waving her hand at me.

"Come here," I see her say. I follow the path—the red, orange, and yellow rocks hot beneath my feet—gold all around me. It vibrates, flickers, and flashes. There is a shimmer and glisten of red behind me and burgundy beneath me. I walk and stars are all around me. They ping, tingle, clang, and click. I hear them snapping, cracking, knocking, and popping. The sounds dart in all directions. They burst and explode.

I am lying very quietly under a huge yellow cottonwood. The air is cold. The breath of winter blows on my face. The yellow cottonwood leaves fall, float gently, and hit the river.

"Wolf. Wolf, are you asleep?"

"No, Old Woman. I'm just resting. Resting in the Fall."

"It's time for you to come to the Grand Council. You must get counsel. You must get up. You must go to the Golden Door. He is here, waiting. Look," she says quickly.

I sit up and look. In the water Dark Eyes holds his arms out. His hair is wet and wild. There are water drops on his beard and mustache.

"Come quickly, Wolf," he says. "You need to get to the Golden Door now, and listen to the Council of Grand. There you will begin to understand your Grandness. I worry about you from time to time, because I don't see respect for your Grandness. When you pass the Golden Door, there will be those who tell you you are Grand."

"Who said I needed to be Grand? Why is it you are making this choice for me?"

"A shaman is Grand," he replies. "And you are in the Grand level of Rainbow Medicine. Are you lost?" He raises his eyebrow and grins.

"No, I'm not lost."

I jump in the water. It's cold. I emerge in his arms and he spins me around, lifting me high and letting me stand on his hand. Then he throws me in the air, way high. I love that about the spirit world—I can fly! I burst upwards, soar, and float down towards him. Slowing, drifting, I fall into his arms.

"One more kiss," I say. "One more, before I go."

He blows softly in my face, and I say, "No. Give me my kiss."

"That is your kiss." He blows and small stars splash from his mouth, burgundy stars, silver stars, white stars, and soft pale blue stars. They fill my hair, and get on my eyebrows. I can feel them and see them standing on the bridge of my nose.

I look in his eyes and before me I see a Golden Door. I hear the tiny voices of the stars that are all over my face, on my arms and my hands, and all over my shirt. They are singing and clapping, "Go now, Wolf, quick. Go now, and open the door."

It is beautiful—solid wood—golden wood. Shimmering, shivering, gold and white light radiates from all edges of the door, beneath and above. As I get closer to the door, I notice an etching. It is that of an Elk Man. It is Dark Eyes.

"Yes," he whispers. "Romance is your mind. I am your heart. Remember your blue heart. Remember the heart of Truth. Remember no matter how mortal we seem, we are not. We are only here. I am your heart."

I feel my heart beating. My soul aches. I feel like weeping desperately. I think of the knife. It is a fading moment, and I hear the voice of Fading Deer. "Don't think of her, don't listen. Remember the elders. You must listen to the elders."

"I can listen to the elders," I say. "But gold—why do I have to go through the Golden Door? Gold is mortal. I don't trust the gold, and I don't want to open a Golden Door." I shake my head.

He looks at me and sighs. "Wolf, we are in the spirit world. You must go through the Golden Door and listen to the wisdom of the golden elders, for they will teach you the Grandness of the world."

"No, no, no," I say. "If I open the door all of the spirit world will disappear!"

"Well, you must not have much spiritual faith. No, I'm not even going to argue with you this time, girl. Just open the door."

"Why?" I say in the best little girl voice I have. "That won't change anything either. This section of the wheel is about maturity."

"Don't worry. I will always be here. I am you." He points at his heart. "Go."

I feel myself enter his very essence. I go deep within his soul.

Colored spiraling stars spin and flash, lighting up everything around me. I feel the ground spinning—and the air spinning; I feel myself spinning—becoming pure energy. Now I am stars. I am beyond. I let go.

"I love you, and you must remember and know that love is being understood," Dark Eyes says. "It is being believed and supported. And most of all it is connected."

Whoosh—the wind spins around me.

Bam! I run into a solid force, right into his huge chest. He is an awesome old one.

"You're here," he says. "I am Winter Ram."

He is standing flat-footed in front of me. I smell his wildness. His face is long and narrow. His hair is long and wild, dark golden brown with streaks of white and gray. He is a physical male, a spiritual ram. His eyes are deep-set, yellow circles with black dots in the center. His chest has long hair. He is enormous.

I step back and look up. Beyond him are grand mountains, covered with snow. I close my eyes softly. When I open them, my eyes are drawn to Winter Ram's belt, where a knife sheath holds a huge bowie knife with a handle made from the Grand Rolled Horn Ram.

"Dark Eyes is right. I am the one who tells you you are Grand." He turns and extends his hand, his finger pointing towards the mountain, thumb up and fingers rolled in. "There. You must fly there, Wolf. You must extend your mind and rise in flight. There you will go to the golden circle—the Council of Grand. Why is it, do you think," he says, closing his eyes softly, "that it is so hard for humans to accept their Grandness?" He opens his eyes and looks at me.

"I don't know, "I say.

"Being Grand is the easiest thing you do," he says. "For it is the you within each of us."

"You?" I say, pointing at him.

"Yes, you." He points back at me. He scoops his hand down and picks me up, and tosses me just a little, gently, like a ball. "I will send you on now for that is my job. You must speak to the Elders, the Council of Grand." He tosses me and I soar.

I fly through the Golden Doorway, and enter into a golden room. It is warm and friendly, like sunlight shining in the window on a happy Sunday morning. I can smell the familiar aromas of coffee and hot chocolate, chicken soup and homemade bread, apples baking, piñon wood burning, cedar, and sage. Entering the room from the right are spirits. They are light spirits, long, willowy cylinders of light. They are very tall. As I watch them, I feel myself getting taller. I rise high and look down. I have the feeling of long arms and thinness.

The first one stands in front of me. His color is a radiant red. It pulsates and changes from shades of light red to deep, rich, blood red. His whole chest is heart. I can see it beating and pulsating. "I am Heart. I have come here to share," the spirit speaks in a deep, radiant voice. "Sit with me and the others and we will speak to you now."

The spirit spins around. Many long spears of glass make up this spirit's hair. It is wild and full, and as he shakes his head, the spikes of glass hit against each other and make sharp sounds. The noise is unbelievably loud—piercing sounds of church bells rattle and clang.

"Feel me, I am Heart. Fire Heart is my name," and he sits.

The next one has no hair. It has no arms, either, only legs—long legs with sharp knees. I look at its orange color as it waves in and out. It makes me dizzy. It pulsates as it waves. The colors moving in the tube are bright and hot orange, very soft and pale orange.

"I am Energy. I am the storyholder. I speak the story of memory. I am the storyholder," and it sits down.

I watch the two spirits, their straight tube-like bodies now quivering like jelly. They move and take form in any way they want.

The yellow spirit announces itself as the brainwaves.

The green one says it is the bone speaker.

The blue one says it is the life force, the blood.

The purple one calls itself the mind.

The last one joins us. It is tall and silent, cold and deep, burgundy in color. It looks at me and says, "I am Spirit."

"If you're Spirit, then part of me is you?" I ask. "And how can I be here and you be there and I be a part of you?"

I hear music—Big Music.

"Hear that?" he says. "It is all us. When you are on earth, everything is separated. That is the birth of words. Here it is all one song."

I become the music and we are all one. I can feel the moving, the warm gentle sway. Each one of the spirits sits; they form a circle around me. I look at them and their faces are all human. I look from left to right and their faces change to animal to human to formless color, to a jiggling, wiggling, Jell-O-like substance, to masses of swirling, colorful fog. I become quiet and limp. I lie down on a blanket that appears for me. The blanket is black with a rainbow-colored raven in the center.

"I speak to you, for I am Heart. I am the spokesman of the Council of

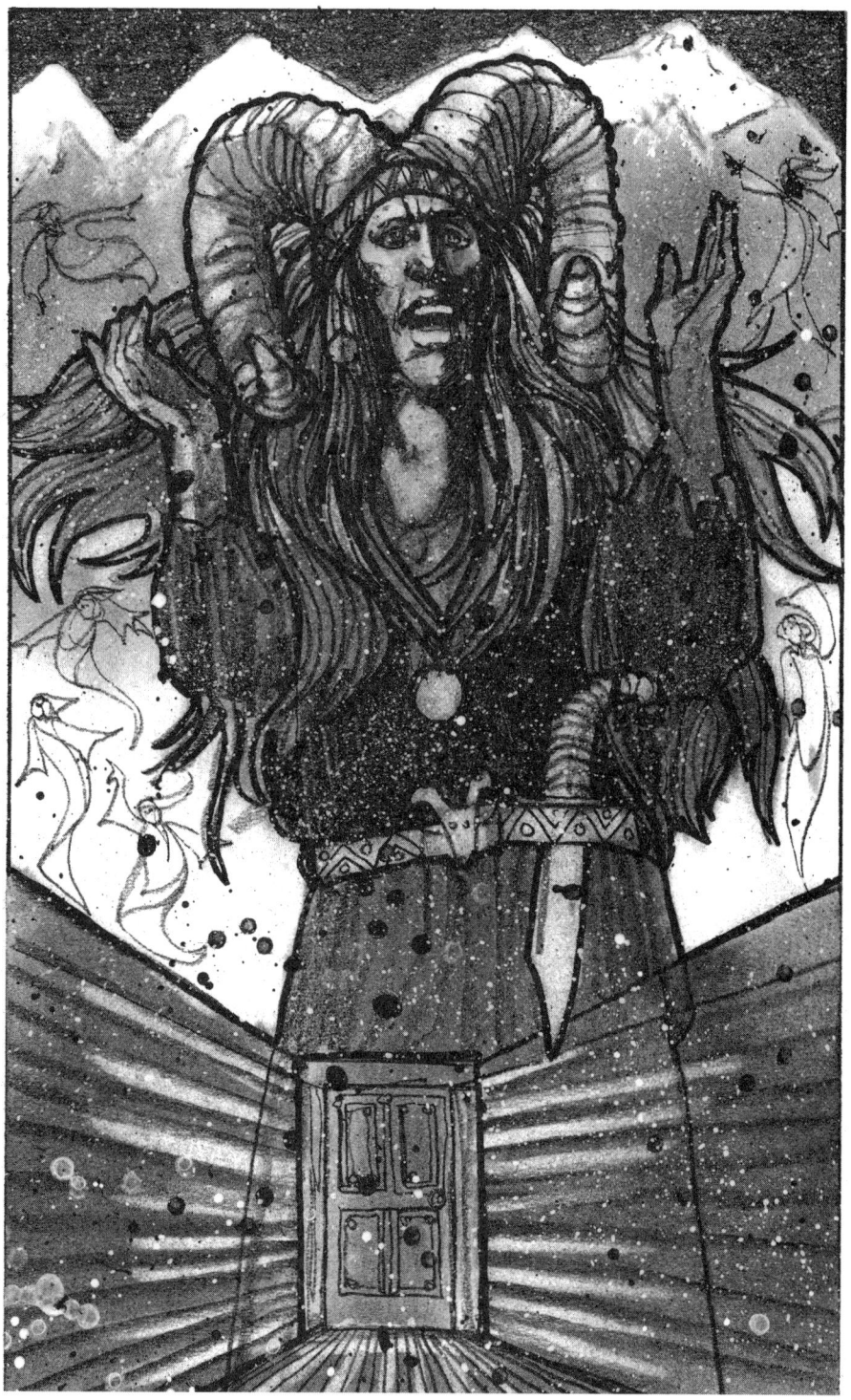

Grand Spirits. You are us and we are all. Because you teach, we share the voice of the sun, the moon, and the seven sacred stars. All begins with color. Colors are the songs. Colors are the healings. Colors are the healers. Colors are the teachers," Spirit speaks.

The others are quiet, shimmering tubes of color that glisten all around me. The room is full of color. It makes sounds, and you can feel the frequencies change, the cracks, pops, and fracturing. All around me is intense. But I am warm, comfortable, and safe on the black raven blanket.

The red spirit takes a breath and speaks again. "Those who call themselves Grand need to be humble. Those who think they are better than others must listen to the lessons and pay their respects to life. For only others can say you are Grand. We have called you here so that there on Earth you remember your spirit. Spirit is burgundy, and burgundy is Grand. We say you are Grand. For you are spirit."

Heart looks at me and says, "We agree that if you ask your students, they will tell you that you are a Grand teacher. We have come to you to tell you to speak the words of color always, for you are our caretaker. You are a carrier of the Grand Council. Remember the spirit who stands tall and guards the mountains? The Grand Ram. You can go to him, and he can take you back through the door—anytime. Or you can teach on, walking the path here within the Grand Council. It is yours within the Big Music to turn back at any time and become a simple mortal. Because that is what humans want to do," the spirit says. Its voice echoes off the walls.

"That's what they want to do," the spirits all say, in clear, cutting tones.

Energy speaks—the orange spirit. "The nervous system can only take so much stress, anger, and denial. Sickness resonates all through the nervous system. That's the big secret to cancer, AIDS, and Alzheimer's. It's the big secret that waits ahead of those who push themselves beyond respect." The voice of the orange spirit grows softer and more pleasant. Then it draws a breath in, and I hear the fracturing of sound and the chiming church bells. The sound seems as if it is going to split my head. I feel as if I am going to be sucked away.

The skeleton begins to speak. "Listen for the caw of the raven. Follow the dark road, come to the tree and turn to the North and walk into the night, and watch for the seven white lights."

The skeleton spirit stands and begins to swirl. It is huge—tall and thin. It begins to dance, moving its arms up and down, taking the form of a spider, raising its pointed knees and pointing its toes down. It dances a raw, wild, Native dance. It dances all around us to a multi-faceted drum beat—a Native percussion of sound.

The spirits all begin to dance. I am so small that, beneath them, I feel like a speck of dust. As they dance, they roll me up in the blanket, wrapping and folding, and spin me up into the air. I fly on the blanket, as if it is a magic carpet.

The blanket floats and flutters; it drifts wide open and lands on the ground. I lie there in peace and quiet, watching the cottonwood glisten above me, glancing at the enormous mountains across the water. I hear the sounds of the wind tinkling and rattling the bones in the tree. I feel the presence of Dark Eyes' love lifting me in his strength. I smell the aromas of home just up the path.

"Who here says she is Grand?" my assistant asks. "Who says she is a Grand Teacher?"

All the students raise their hands. There is applause.

"Once more, Wolf Moondance completes your studies," she says, "and you students are free to go."

"I will look forward to seeing you in two weeks," I tell them, "for then you will hear the call of the Wolf."

I hear the rattling of the bones calling me back.

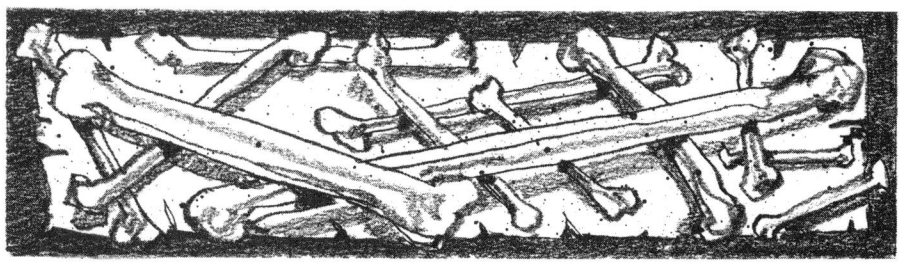

Teachings of Grand—Ram Medicine

What makes a Grand warrior? What makes a Grand teacher? What makes your Grandmother and your Grandfather? It has to be the things they do, what they worship and where they go to church, how much education they have, how smart they are, and how much money they have—right? I have a unique and plain definition of Grand that I live with. When you seek out a Grand one, he or she has the right to bestow upon you your Grandness by asking others, "Who here thinks this person is Grand?"

It doesn't matter how long you live your life, how many diplomas you have, how much money you have made or spent, how many things you own, how many countries you have visited, or how many hands you have shaken—that have shaken the hand that shook the hand of the hand that shook the hand...

It isn't about being in the vicinity that makes you Grand. Grand is a sacred society of worth, and worth is bestowed upon you through humbleness. Sometimes you are born humble and sometimes you have to be humbled. Sometimes you are born exuberant, powerful, and important. You are revered and splendid; you are total, stately, and complete. When that happens, I like to call it the curse of Grandness. I used to take my Grandness lightly, and I used to think it was a curse. I used to think that what was important was being popular, with everyone wanting to come over to your house, for example, when I was in school. Then I realized that I had a tremendous responsibility to respect, to organization, to dedication, to beauty, and to life itself, to be called Grand.

We often look into the wilderness and think of the elk, the wolf, the grizzly bear, and the bald eagle, and call them majestic and Grand. The true teaching of Grand is knowing the Grand ones when you see them. They will be gentle, forgiving, wise, calm. The Grand one will see your self-Nurture, see your right Choices, and know that you are one who performs Ceremony. The Grand one will know that you make Changes and that you are Real. When the Grand one, or anyone in your presence, sees your Proof as Grandness, you are truly Grand.

So when you envy others and think that they're Grand, it's probably the other way around—that they know that you're Grand and they aren't sure that you know they even exist.

To obtain your Grandness and find out if you are, here is a small Ceremony of Grandness that I ask you to do for yourself.

Ceremony of Grandness

TOOLS: *Journal and pen to take notes on your adventure of Grandness.*

Seek out seven people and ask them to tell you what, if anything, is Grand about you. Grandness is defined as impressive, stately, ambitious, revered, important, complete, and excellent. Ask them these questions and write down their answers.

> What do I do that is impressive?
> What is stately about me?
> What am I ambitious about?
> Why am I revered by you?
> Why am I important to you?
> What do you see about me that is complete?
> What do I do that is excellent in your eyes?

When the seven people answer these questions, you can look and see if they know you or not. If they speak of the quality of your hair, the quality or sound of your voice, your kindness, your committedness, your loyalty, your spirituality, your reverence, and your sincerity—then you can honor yourself as a truly worthy warrior. You can honor yourself as a Grand teacher. You can feel good within yourself in a humble way, that you reflect the image that you are made of, our Great Spirit, our Grand Creator, our God.

If you are made in the image of God then I would say that you are Grand.

If you fail the test because you cannot find seven people, or if you find seven people and fail the test because they can't think of anything Grand about you, then the first thing I suggest is that you find different people! If you can't find people, I recommend that you get counseling to find out why you stifle yourself, why you have self-rage and an urge to self-destruction.

As we walk with our medicine of Grandness, it opens our opportunities to heal the brokenness, the emptiness, the fearfulness of being human.

Aho.

Shaman's Necklace

A shaman's necklace is brought forth to empower you, to physically represent the teachings of Bone Medicine at all the different levels and in all the teachings of the seven colors within Rainbow Medicine. When you bring about a shaman's necklace it is your Choice to make it how you want it to be. I am setting the theme for this shaman's necklace, as the shaman overseeing this project. Each teacher, each spiritualist, each visionary, each medicine person that you work with, might want you to carry a shaman's necklace made the way he or she recommends it.

Often, a shaman's necklace is a pouch. Protection pouches, which are small skin pouches that carry objects you draw strength from, are a very popular way of wearing a shaman's necklace. Another way is simply to wear an article that represents your animal totem, such as a wolf's tooth, a badger claw, or horsehair. The object represents the power that you gain from your shamanic animal guide.

The medicines within your shaman's necklace are the teachings of Bone Medicine. They are the Nurture, Choice, Ceremony, Change, Proof, Real, and Grand medicines that you have encountered in these writings. You can also look in the back of the book in the Color section and connect other words to your shaman's necklace—words that are in the color definitions. It is a good thing to wear your shaman's necklace at all times when you are doing spiritual work or trying to achieve something where you need to feel empowered, physically, through the connection of your spirit.

TOOLS: *Gold and silver embroidery thread, or a strong gold and silver cord or wire, so that you can string your objects and wear them as a necklace; clay, which you can purchase at a craft store, and which you can form and make into certain objects, if you wish; beads, that represent the words of the West section of the medicine wheel; beads that represent the depth of the teachings of each word within the West section; beads or objects that represent your personal self; pen and journal; ceremonial herb supplies for smudging; a quiet place, and your blanket.*

When you are making your shaman's necklace, find a quiet place where you can work with the seven words in the West section known as Bone Medicine. Sit and think about what Nurture means to you, what Choice means to you, what Ceremony means to you—what each word within the section means to you—and journal these thoughts.

Example: *In my shaman's necklace, I have a sun that represents the directions, a star for each word, and the moon that represents wisdom. Between them I have a black and white bead that represents spirit and physical.*

When you are making your shaman's necklace, you only need seven objects or seven beads to represent the seven words of the West section of the Medicine Wheel. If you wish to make your necklace larger and have it represent other words from the color guides, then feel free to connect several words to each color, bringing forth several beads to represent the teachings. Between each section you can apply your own personal bead, so that you will have a personal bead—then the red section; a personal bead—then the orange section; a personal bead—then the yellow section, all the way to the burgundy section, followed by a personal bead. Give yourself enough cord to add a hook, so you can fasten your necklace and wear it when you need to.

When you have strung your necklace, it is individual to you. You may choose to use objects such as bones from animals, teeth, things that are made from clay, objects that are stone, or carved fetishes. It is up to you how you want to make your shaman's necklace. Remember that your shaman's necklace should be kept in a pouch or wrapped in red cloth when you are not wearing it. Place it on your altar or in another sacred place where you keep your special objects in your home. I recommend that it be respected; that it not be an object of sale. You cannot sell it; it cannot be traded; and it is passed on only to your own children. If you choose to give another a shaman's necklace, then you can make it for them, and empower it with the words that you wish to give them.

When you are wearing your shaman's necklace, it is important to remember that it is there to help you with your Grandness, to give you your Grandness, and show you—through your own spirit and listening to the words as medicines—how to produce great accomplishments in your life. When you are finished making your shaman's necklace, put all your tools away, and put it on. Enjoy it as you walk your life, listening to its teachings.

Aho.

Process of the Lesson of Worthy—Lynx Teachings

The lynx sits quietly beside the tree. It blends in with the snows, the pale Fall grasses, and with the new grass in the snow of the Spring. It fits in the Summer with its brownness. The lynx keeps its secrets, as we do with our worth.

The lesson is to obtain the secrets of our worth, to understand that our worth is our spirit. If we are spirited, then we are truly worthy—we are rich, full, and intense.

When we think of Great Spirit, Creator, God—we see the power of creation. When we look at death, we see the intensity of Change. When we study the human brain, we are faced with the intensity of our thought. Our worth is just as intense. Knowing our worth, and showing it quietly in our daily walk, we demonstrate worthy.

That is why it is necessary to have a Ceremony of Worth.

Ceremony of Worthy

TOOLS: *Burgundy candle and holder; 14 stones; 13 pillows or pads for people to sit on; 12 people you know who will come together in a circle and speak of your worthiness; a journal and pen; 13 pieces of paper and 13 pens or pencils; a place to come together, to sit and talk; matches to light the candle; smudge sage and bowl.*

1. Find a place where you can gather 12 people in a circle. Lay 13 pads or pillows down, including one for yourself. In the Ceremony of Worthy, invite 12 people to come and speak about your worthiness and your worth. Invite people who you believe will express their feelings truthfully. They don't have to know you; they just have to be willing to speak about what you are worth. Knowing you doesn't change what they will say about your being worthy.

2. Set the room by smudging it and yourself before you start. Place the burgundy candle in the center of the circle, and put 14 stones in a circle around the bottom of the candle—one for each lesson and each medicine in the medicine wheel. Make a circle of the stones around the candle. Then light the candle.

3. Have all the people sit in the circle. Hand them each a paper and pen

and ask them to write down what your worth is, how they see you as a worthy person. Have them complete their papers and pass them to you.

4. After you have obtained their feelings on paper, have them share aloud what they have written about you. Do not be embarrassed by what they say, for it is their statement of worth and worthiness. If they say that you are not worthy, or that you are not of any worth, that is not what you asked them, and you can say that if they start to speak negatively. But I feel it is always good to let people speak their minds, because then they have had their day in court. What they say does not make you who you are. It is simply a balancing point for you to evaluate other people's feelings about your presence and then formulate your truths.

5. Listen to all comments and say thank you.

6. Listen for key words like weak, irresponsible, reliable, inadequate, intelligent, ignorant, selfish. These key words are the building blocks of your worthiness. When they have finished and you have listened to your key words, ask yourself if they are what you wish to be worth.

> **Example:** *One person might say that you are a responsible parent. Ask yourself if that is a goal in your life, to be a responsible parent. Another person might say that you are an inconsiderate, selfish human being. Ask yourself if that has been a goal in your life, to be seen as being inconsiderate and selfish. If it is, then you are a success.*

7. When you are finished, remember that this seventh question is a hard one, but it is how you learn and grow and achieve your Grandness. Ask who in the circle thinks you are Grand. Have them raise their hands. If all 12 say you are Grand, you are Grand. If even one person says no, then you need to look at their worth statement and see where your weaknesses are in their eyes. At that moment, you need to look within your own self—at your goals and purposes—and see if that is how you mean to represent yourself.

Ask what you can do to fix your worth in their eyes. Ask them to select a lesson word from the section of the Medicine Wheel you are studying, so you can learn from it. Choose from purpose, obedience, life, action, solid, full, and worthy.

After you have dismissed the people from the circle and put away everything used in the ceremony, sit with the burgundy candle and ask yourself about your relationship with each person you invited. Ask yourself the reason for the relationship, and whether you respect each person's boundaries and needs. If you have acceptance and understanding for the relationship, but the person sees no worth in you—and you accept the fact that it is not a healthy relationship for you and is beyond repair—you can let the relationship go.

Next are the actions you will take connected to each statement that you have journaled.

Actions

1. Are you willing to stand solid and seek out counseling if you find that you have no worth in anyone's eyes?

2. Are you willing to accept and admit your mistakes or that you are angry and need counseling?

3. Are you able to sit with your own spiritual guides, your shamanic journeys, and the lessons of the Rainbow Medicine Wheel and put yourself in order, so that you can take counsel from your appropriate friends, your appropriate family members, and colleagues?

4. Are you able to sit with yourself, and from the lessons you have learned in life and the applications of your medicines, know what is Grand about yourself and what is not? Use personal affirmations that you like, especially ones that make you laugh.

After looking over all of the statements and asking yourself the Action questions, finish with the last set of questions:

1. Do you know how to set boundaries so that you are able to bring light and goodness to your life, so that you would not harm another or bring harm to yourself?

2. Would you move on and stay away from those who see no worth in you and understand that you have self worth and declare your worth?

3. Would you accept that you don't have to change, that you are who you are and who you want to be?

4. And finally, would you forgive yourself for feeling that you are an unworthy person?

When you look at the lesson of worthy, it is important to understand that you must accept your weaknesses and your shortcomings as expectations of others. The only time you have weaknesses and shortcomings is when you have set goals for your own personality. To obtain your self worth, you must understand that life is made of choices and that you walk in your strength and your truth. You must understand that in the medicine wheel, the crossbars, the cross that you carry in life, is that you live your lessons. It is important to understand that when you point your finger at other people and say that they are the reason that you have a fault, you are in denial and can't accept your own faults.

Often in life people do things that are their fault. But it is your fault that you have not left them and closed the door behind you. Never give your power to another to cast judgment on you.

As you go to blow out your Grand burgundy candle, sit with the beauty of your burgundy stone in Grandness and say to yourself that your worth is the image of Great Spirit. Ask yourself what does Great Spirit look like to you, and be that in your earth walk.

Aho.

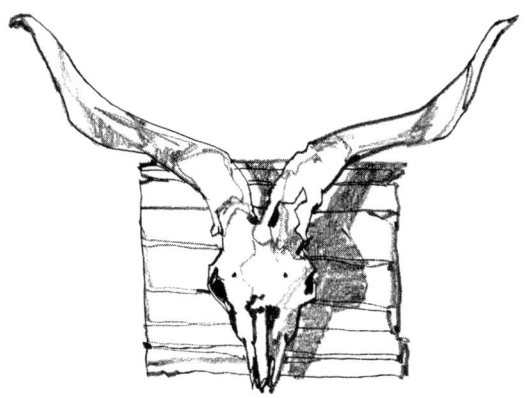

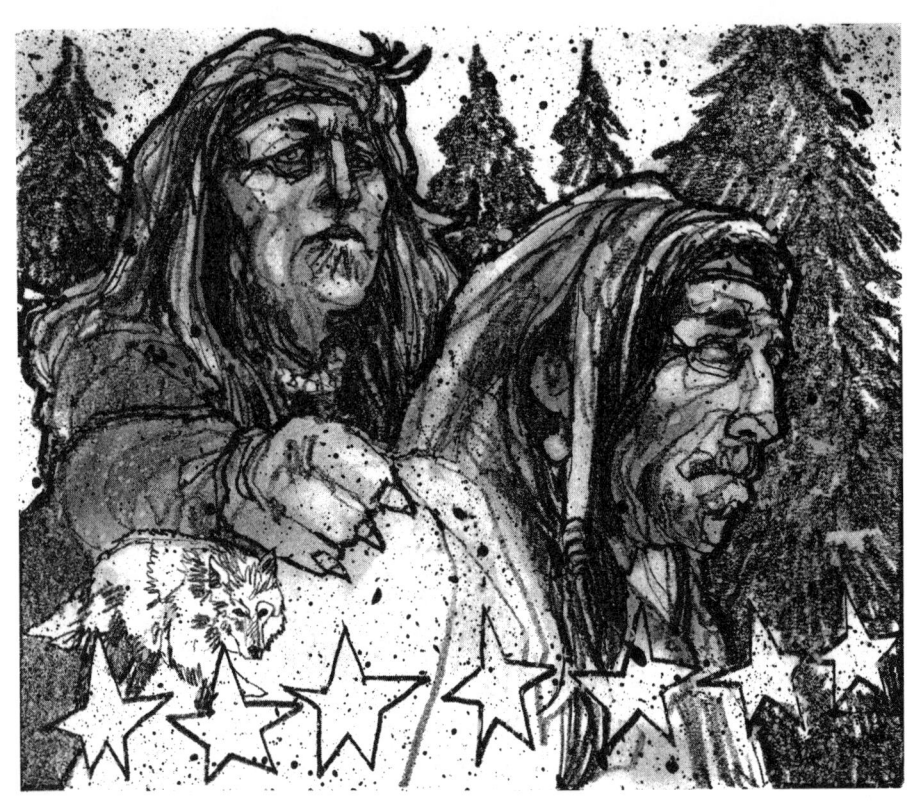

10
THE CALL OF THE WOLF

I breathe in and out four times, softly. I am sitting at the Medicine Wheel in the North, on a stump by the gate. It is early Winter. I feel the cold all around me. Far away in the distance I hear a howling, the cry of a wolf. I hear the coyotes answering it, and I can't help but think of King Coyote, knowing that he holds human beings imprisoned in their own emotions, playing games with them, taunting them, making fun of them, causing anger to rise. I can't help but honor him as a Grand teacher of trickery. It must be an incredible experience, though, King Coyote, to sit there cloaked in all your greenness and emotions, advertising yourself as innocence and growth. I stare across at the green flag on the South gate, a bitter taste in my mouth, thinking of the sharp fingernails that dug into Dark Eyes' shoulders.

A soft, fresh snow is falling. I see a pathway before me. It is a path of footprints in the snow and I begin to follow it. I walk deep into the woods. I hear the call of the wolf again, the howling, piercing sound. Up a-ways in a clearing I see the teepee, sitting quietly, nestled in the woods. The fire inside it glows and smoke is spiraling from the top.

I follow the footprints.

From the right of me comes an old one, running and screaming. "Get out of here," she cries with a quivering voice. "Go on. I don't want you around here. I've heard of you!" She is carrying a stick, and she shakes it at me. "Haven't you people caused me enough pain anyhow? Leave! I live out here on the edge. I don't need anybody telling me what to do. Get on out of here."

She draws a large knife from the side of her skirt and swings it around like a crazy woman. She is getting closer, a wild look on her face. Her ratty hair is all tangled.

"Yeah, that's right." She stops right in front of me. A large figure—almost six feet tall—she is big-boned, with an old saggy face and no teeth. Her eyes are inflamed.

She is dressed in all different kinds of cloth that she has hand-sewn together to make a skirt. Her top is made from two or three different types of blouses that she has ripped and torn up. She has sewn on one sleeve from one blouse, the other from another; one side of the front is one blouse, the other side is another. She has some barbed wire wrapped around her waist, and in it she has stuck several types of sticks and twigs, with bundles of grass and herbs hanging on it like a belt. She wears a backpack full of sticks. She is scruffy and dirty. She is repulsive.

"Whatcha staring at? This is mine. I stole it. Yeah, I took it down from the Cheyenne River people. I stole it from them when they were in Real time. They weren't paying no attention, so I just jerked it up in my mind and I brought it here so I can live in their house. I like them teepees," she says. She has a southern drawl and a staggering depth in her voice—gruff, growly, alcoholic. "And I drink that alcohol," and she spits chewing tobacco right on my foot. "I've been awaiting on you. They call you the Grand Teacher back there on the Earth Mother. They don't call you that here. You're just another one of my students here," and she spits again.

She is breathing fiercely, swinging her knife in a circle in front of me. "I need you to get on out of here, but I want you to look at something, too." She points towards a post that is sticking in the ground. There is a head stuck on the post.

I look at it. "I sure hope that's not a human head."

"Well, what do you think it is," she says. "What do you think I'd stick on that pole?"

"You cut heads off?"

"I cut hair off, I cut heads off, I cut arms and legs off. I'll cut your heart out if you stand there long enough! Now get on out of here!"

Fire shoots from her eyes, and her features become monstrous. She has sores all over her face. Blood is dripping from the right side of her head. I close my eyes and take a big deep breath of cold air. Standing behind her teepee now are five colored horses—a black one, a turquoise one, a pearl-colored one, a red one, and a white one.

"Don't you be getting no ideas about my horses," she says. "My name is Stick Woman, anyhow. I guess they call you Whitey, huh?"

"No, my name is Wolf," I say. "Wolf Moondance."

"Oh yeah. Yeah, that's right. White Wolf Woman. I know you that way. You know me. I'm the one who sees like you do. I see them hurt the children when I'm peeking in there. I go down into town and I peek in there, and I see what they do to the children. I know what they do, because they did it to me. They hurt me and they drove me out here. Now they say I'm bad after they hurt me. I'm out of my mind, that's what I am. You know they say the same thing about you."

She takes her hand and wipes it across her mouth and slings spit on the ground with chewing tobacco in it. "They say things about you, you know. That's why your Grandmother and Grandfather Wolf have sent you here. You see that gateway over there with that white flag a-blowing on it? That there is where you have to go next. That there is where you are going to go, and you're going to see the mind. There is only one who can help you and that's the Blue-Eyed Raven."

I hear the call of the Raven. There is a clicking sound and I see him sitting in the tree above her house.

"Yeah, he's a friend of mine. He's the only one who hasn't ever said that I'm crazy and you know he could. The Raven, he knows the magic of the mind. You'd like him back down there on the Earth Mother. You'd be a good couple. You can forget all these days of Dark Eyes and

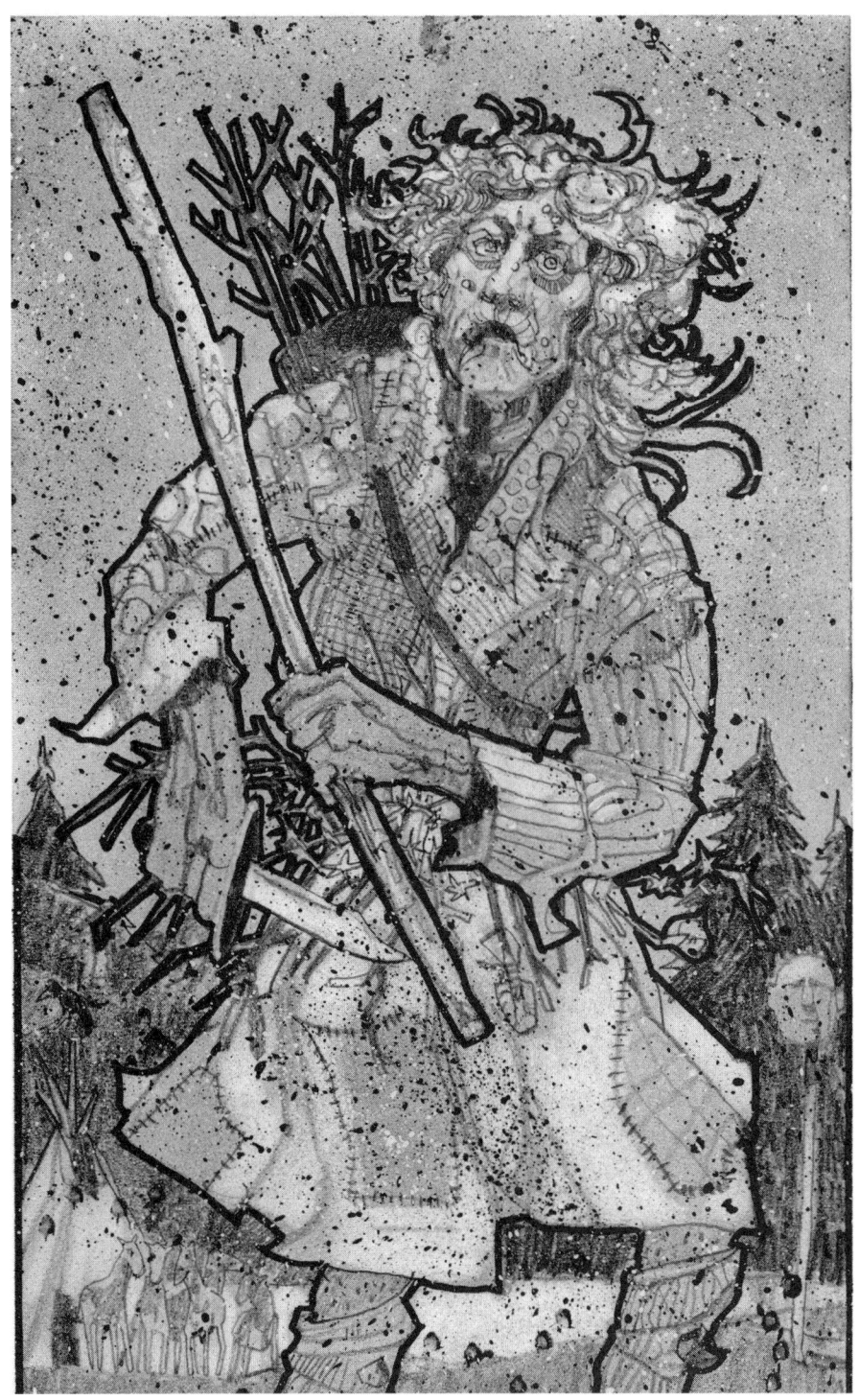

all the dreams and the lollygagging around you've been doing here in the body. 'Cause them days are coming to an end 'cause you're going to understand him and you're going to know where you've been around this circle. That's you, you know. You go around your Medicine Wheel, whoever you are. I see them doing their medicine circles and the medicine dances."

She looks at me with hate in her eyes. I see the scars on the side of her face, places where she has been cut with knives and they've stitched it up—places where it looks like someone hit her with a whip and she has big swollen marks. She slobbers on herself when she speaks. Oh, my heart goes out to her. She is a sad, baggy-looking thing.

"Don't be feeling sorry for me, 'cause I can hear you thinking. You're going to want to come in that house there. You're going to want to stay with me. Well, I want you to understand something: Everything hanging there—even my polecat—it's all mine. I like to hang stuff up there. That's okay though, 'cause they talk about you. Everybody talks about you—Great Teacher, the spiritual one, the Shaman. You walk in two worlds. I do too. I walk in the world of pain," she says with a snarl in her voice. "I walk there in them streets and I used to be one of them. I used to go to church with them. But no, I'm out here now. That's okay. The Raven knows. He listens to me." She draws a deep, wheezing breath and spits another hunk of tobacco on the ground. "Come on," and she starts walking towards the tepee. She sort of waddles and limps.

What unique horses! I've never seen a red horse before.

"Don't be thinking about them things. Just get on up here and come in. Got to get you up a bed before that Winter wind gets any stronger tonight. You'd better bring in some of them bundles of sticks," and she points her long, skinny finger towards a wood pile of neatly stacked and tied sticks. "Go get some and earn your keep. Bring them on in, and I'll stir up the possum soup, and we'll have some."

She goes inside. I am walking towards the sticks and trying to get over the sight of the head that was stuck on the pole. I decide maybe I'll get a little closer and take a look. The closer I get the more I notice. It has a face, and that face is washed out white. But the head is a pumpkin! The old woman has taken a pumpkin, painted its face white, and cut out its eyes, nose, and mouth. A candle is burning in it, just like a jack-o-lantern ought to have, and some moss is stuck on to make hair.

Stick Woman's deep, rough voice echoes in my mind. What a disgusting creature! I gather up the bundles of wood and head back to the tepee. I lift the skin flap and step inside. The smell almost knocks me back out.

"Yeah, everybody always thinks the mind is so pretty. They always think everything smells good. Ain't nothing smells good in the body. This here is the earth and it's dead. It's rotten, rotted, foul-smelling, dead things—that's what the earth is. Winter is death, you know. That's White Face out there. Winter. This here is my sacred house, and they say you're going to be staying here with me. Over there is your bed," and she points her old finger to the floor and a pile of buffalo skins.

It's getting cold, and the wind is whistling around the tepee, but she has the bottom of it packed in tight with grasses and sticks. In the center of the floor, a tripod is set over the fire, and a pot hangs from the tripod. I look in the pot and say, "Is this one of those spiritual stews?"

"Nah, it's just plain old possum. I found it dead out there and I cut it up and cooked it, threw some roots in, and it'll be good for you. You do eat these spiritual things here, but I want you to know that I'm an earth walker. Ain't nothing nice about me 'cause I'm crazy, you see."

She gives a big sniff and draws her arm across and wipes the snot off her nose. She gets this funny, glassy look in her eyes and just kind of stares off over my shoulder. I turn and see a dark silhouette passing across the wall of the tepee. I sense the presence of Darkness, and it feels good to be in the old woman's home.

"Yeah, I can be, though. They say insane is real crazy. You know, those people who don't understand mental. Us mentals, we're all the same. You know, they're scared of us. They call us retards and rejects, and they say we're psychotic. Well, I ain't no psychotic. I ain't no mental case neither."

I notice that her right eye twitches and it is drawn in, and her left eye is big.

"You looking at that? Yeah, that's what my daddy did when I was three. He loved me a lot, poked my eye right out of there."

I see a white ball where the eyeball should be. How could anybody be so mean to a child?

"It's easy. You know it, White Wolf Woman. You know. Oh, Wolf Moondance knows broken bones, don't you? You know the anguish of the mind when you've been hurt unfairly."

173

She reaches down and pitches a rolled-up blanket towards me. "You're going to need that there with those bearskins too, 'cause it's going to get cold in here. It won't get cold in our beds, though, 'cause we're comfortable here. I promised your Grandfather Wolf I'd take real good care of you. It's going to be a while before you be hearing him and Grandmother again here in the mind. You've got some things to hear and listen to. Stick Woman, I'll be right here with you. I'll be Grandmother. I'll help you. I won't leave you unattended. Nobody will be hurting you."

I take my knife and cut the straps she has tied on the blanket. It is a beautiful red wool blanket with a Sioux star in the center—an eight-pointed star. It has been rubbed and wrapped in sage and it smells real good.

I say, "Old Woman, I'm awful tired. I'm feeling like I'm going to just go to sleep now."

"Oh, you ain't sleeping none. You've got to have some of this here stew now, don't you?"

"No, no." I say, putting my gear beside the mat of skins. I lie down on the bear rug, and cover up with the blanket. I listen to the song of the wind outside the tepee, and watch the fire in the center swirl around under the pot of stew. She gets up and hunkers over it, belches a couple of times, puts a big dipper of it in her cup, and sits down. She starts sucking and smacking, chewing, and slurping.

Oh, I can't hardly wait to walk to seven medicine stones plus seven lessons with her!

Oh, I breathe a sigh of relief, because I'm beginning to get warm. My mind drifts to the sky, and it is white. All around me are black, shiny, twinkling stars with blue dots in the center. The stars look like blue eyes watching me.

As I lie there and listen to her eat, I think about how mean people can be, how their Choices in their physical existence can literally destroy the minds of others.

"Hey, Old Woman, I bet the river is pretty this time."

"Eh, you're a long way from the river," she says. "You ain't going to be getting up that way. You're going to come to an understanding that you don't need to be thinking of your childhood things, 'cause that ain't going to do you no good. You're going to come to a spot where you understand that the smile of the bobcat is where the secrets are."

Great, I think to myself.

I reach into my medicine pouch and pull out Dark Eyes' blue-faceted heart. I remember his gentleness and how he said he is always with me.

"Yeah, he's with you," she says and sort of cackles. "Yeah, he's with you. He's just a fantasy you made up so you can handle all the pain. How's it feel, being human? How's it feel being a two-legged?"

I hear the rattling of the bones calling me back.

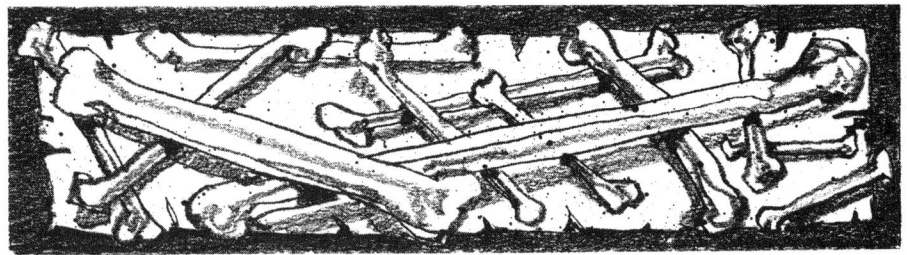

Ceremony of the Five Colored Horses

The mind is within the physical. It is housed in the brain. The mental is the voice of the brain. It is the neurological action that gives us our opportunities, our abilities, and our physical response to spiritual essence. In the Ceremony of the Five Colored Horses, you will experience the horse of the physical bone, the horse of opportunity, the horse of protection, the horse of dreamtime, and the horse of ceremony. The horses will help you find your physical color, locate your opportunities, and work in dreamtime. The horse of the night will help you learn what ceremony to use to solve a situation.

The Ceremony of the Five Colored Horses helps strengthen your understanding of your physical self by connecting you to dreamtime. Dreamtime is the space between the spirit world and the physical world, a place in spirit where you go to learn lessons and proofs about lessons from your spirit guides. It's important to remember that in dreamtime you can feel physical repercussions from the lessons you are learning, such as bruises, scrathes, scrapes, and other physical blemishes. Dreamtime could be called an altered state of consciousness, or being in a trance.

TOOLS: *Candles—turquoise, white, red, pearl (any off-white candle can be used), black; safe candle holders; journal and pen; cornmeal; Ceremony of the Sacred Herbs supplies; medicine blanket.*

Find a quiet place where you will not be disturbed. Lay out your medicine blanket, with your journal and pen, your smudge bowl, and candles. Draw a cornmeal circle around your medicine blanket and step in from the East. Sit comfortably with your journal and pen.

1. The Pearl Horse—the Horse of the Physical Bone

Breathe in and out four times, and relax. Before you, you will see a clear piece of ground, a pasture. The sky is blue and the grass is green. Look around and you will see a pearl-colored horse. This horse is a pale off-white color, a mixture of all colors. When you see the horse, walk up carefully, grab its mane, and pull yourself onto its back. The horse will carry you on a spirit ride. You will be riding deep into yourself. You will come to a creek that runs across the road. Get off the horse and look into the water. There you will see the physical color of your bone (your form). You will see this color very clearly. When you have seen the color, bring it back and write about it in your journal. The color that you have seen in the water of the creek is your clan color.

2. Sunrise—the Red Horse of Opportunity

Breathe in and out deeply four times, and relax. Continue breathing and in front of you, you will see a path on which you are walking in the dawn. You will come to a place where the sky is very clear, and you see the colors of the sunrise. In this beautiful morning setting, you turn and see a red horse. You go to the horse, and recognize it as the horse of opportunity. You grab hold of the horse's mane, pull yourself up on the horse's back, and the horse will carry you on a spirit ride. You come to where the trail ends and look out over a vast, open space. There you are shown your physical opportunities. You will see them very clearly. They might be your physical ability to be healthy; they may be opportunities for jobs, or opportunities within your family. Look very carefully and you will see your physical opportunity. It may come to you in symbols, so bring back what you have seen and record it in your journal, knowing that you can interpret the symbols later.

3. Noon—the Turquoise Horse, the Horse of Protection

You breathe in and out deeply, and relax. Before you, you see a path. It leads you to an old barn. Outside of that barn in the pasture stands a turquoise horse. You walk to the horse, and grab it by its mane. Get on the horse and take a spirit ride. The horse will carry you along the ocean. It is very sunny. You look out across the ocean, and there you have a vision of yourself. Your life's physical weaknesses will be revealed to you, so you can draw upon the energy of the turquoise horse to protect you. You will see the weak parts of yourself—the parts of your physical life that need to be strengthened and nurtured. You will see the physical parts of yourself that need to be protected: It might be a weakness in a bone; it might be a sickness in the body; it might be a bad habit. Remember what you have seen, bring it back, and record it in your spirit journal.

4. Sunset—the Black Horse of Dreamtime

You breathe deeply in and out four times, and relax. You will see before you a path that has white rocks on it. You walk along the road. There in front of you is a black horse that looks directly at you. You look deep into the horse's eyes and you are taken to dreamtime. Deep in the horse's eyes you see the path that helps you find and connect with your spiritual and physical dreamtime. Pay attention to what your path looks like. It might run along the ocean; it might run through the woods; it might run through a garden. It is important for you to connect with your dreamtime path, a place where you can connect with your spirit guides and learn your lessons. Remember the path, bring it back, and record it in your journal.

5. Night—the White Horse of Ceremony

Breathe deeply in and out four times, and relax. Before you, everything is very quiet and still. It is night. There is a silvery white full moon. You see a path of stone that leads through the night. You follow the path and along the way you are approached by a beautiful white horse. You grab hold of the white horse's mane and go for a ride. The horse will take you along the path to an area where ceremonies are taking place. There you will see the ceremony that is necessary for the moment you called for it. The ceremony could be that of marriage, death, healing, joy, sisterhood, brotherhood, freeing the soul, etc. Look carefully at the ceremony that is being performed for you in the clearing. Remember who and what you see, and what they do. Bring it back and record it in your spirit journal.

Use the Horse of the Physical Bone when you need to work with the identity of your physical color. Use the Horse of Opportunity when you need to locate your opportunities. Use the Black Horse when you need a path to enter into dreamtime. Use the horse named Night when you need to call upon a ceremony and learn what ceremony you need to use to solve a situation.

Ceremony of the White Wolf

TOOLS: *A white lunch sack or paper bag; a box of salt; a bag of rock salt; your journal and pen, ceremony of the Sacred Herbs supplies.*

1. As with every ceremony, use your sacred herbs to cleanse your aura.

2. Dump your table salt and the rock salt into a white paper sack. Hold the sack in your hand and know that the ceremonial salt is the white wolf.

3. Open your journal and write down the things that you are afraid of. Think about all of your existence, anything that you have fears about —any earthly fears, any past life fears, soul loss fears, or weaknesses in the self. Write those things down in your journal.

4. When you have brought together all the things you feel might weaken or distress you, take a handful of salt for each one and place it at a point around your house—a special place where you want this salt to build a barrier between you and those weaknesses. You can do this ceremony inside or outside your house. You can lay your salt in either place. When doing a ceremony inside, place the salt under your bed and in front of your doorways by putting a small thin line of it on the floor. When doing the ceremony outside, place a small pile of salt at the four corners of your house and under each window and door.

5. As you place your mound of salt, envision a beautiful white wolf

becoming your friend. Turn that wolf loose to roam the circle of your home, to keep you safe. Know that when you go to rest, your mind will relax and your mental pathways will heal; your old habits will yearn to be dismissed. Think of a habit that you want to release, and let it go by giving it to the salt, by allowing the white wolves to have it for dinner.

6. Wake up in the morning and ask yourself if that habit is still yours. If it is, do the ceremony over again until you no longer have the habit. When you put your feet on the bed for the night, give thanks for your guardian white wolves that watch over you and protect you while you are here as a two-legged taking your test of life.

7. Close your ceremony by putting everything away and being grateful and knowing that you are protected.

Aho.

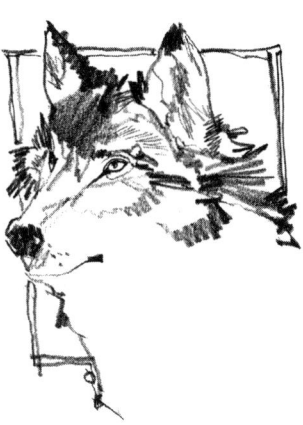

RAINBOW TOTEM AND GUIDE TEACHINGS

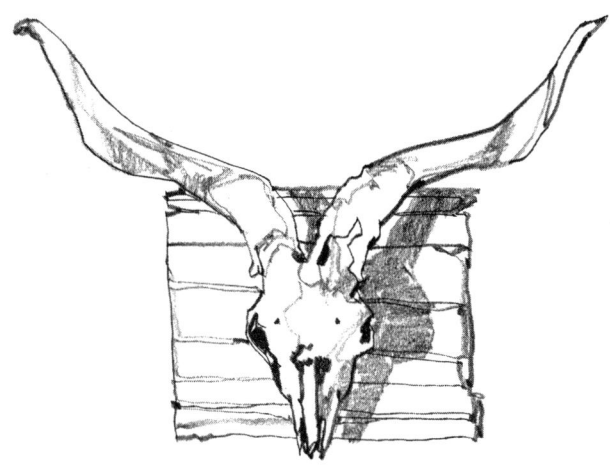

MEDICINE WORDS

Nurture—Red. Nurture is applied confidence. It is the reality of Strength. As applied confidence, it is extended energy. The extending of energy is strength. That type of strength, within Nurture, is a key component in power. Nurture is knowing your path: it is your belief, your faith. Extended energy is maintaining; it is having, as in a teaching or knowing, as in your talent. Applied principles within Nurture are to maintain, cherish, guide, discipline, and teach. To have Nurture is to have a safe space to breathe.

Choice—Orange. Choice is two-sided. Those two sides allow you to draw from your spirit or your physical. In color energy, that would be black or white, silver, or gold. Choice is the point. Choice is choosing, voice, discernment, and embracement.

Choice is spiritual; Choice is physical. The embracement is the physical of Choice; discernment is the spiritual of Choice. Choice is the voice in the fact that it is the path. There is hope within Choice. In choosing, you face the path—a path that is two-sided, physical and spiritual.

Ceremony—Yellow. Ceremony is the physical action of Vision. It is service, strictness, formalities. Creativity has eyes and sees Vision. Vision is a form known as Ceremony, within the formalities of applied respect, honesty, sincerity, and the act of service. Ceremony is a movement that allows you to step into Change.

Change—Green. To Change is to alter, to alter is to do. Ceremony brings about the movement of Choice and propels it into movement. Change is a shift brought about from intention, whose action is do. Change transposes and transforms, which is the metamorphosis of Proof. The actual movement of Change is applied action. In plain words, do it!

Proof—Blue. Proof is one of the more spiritual realities in life. It is validation. It is the mirror of evidence. Physicality is the Proof of the spiritual. Proof allows you to be sure. Proof deepens itself through the Absolute. It is the gateway to Real.

Real—Purple. Real is a total circle—a spiritual given as well as a physical fact. Within the sacred circle of Real, there is fantasy, spiritual, and reality. They meet as a council and come to an agreement, and that is known as Real. Real brings forth actual, factual, realistic, and simple. Our visioning, hoping, dreaming, our acting, are all movements of pure and valid. Real is.

Grand—Burgundy. Grand is achievable by others. It is admitting your immortality, understanding that it is bestowed upon you—that you do not own it. You cannot hold Grand; you can only be Grand. Grand is illusive; it is gentle and enormous. Grand is obtainable through impeccability, through greatness. Through the grace of others you are Grand. It is simple and smooth, difficult and easy. Grand is a level of physicality that is spiritual. It is the reason for existence.

LESSON WORDS

Purpose—Red. Purpose is identity. It is structure, boundaries, limits, understanding, principles, mortality, virtue, and character. Your purpose is your point. It is your expansion in life.

Obedience—Orange. Obedience can be an order or it can be a prayer. It can be direct, or it can be evasive, but to achieve obedience you must recognize that obedience is an order. It is given to you by someone else. Obedience is something that you give to a higher presence, not to other people—unless you bestow upon them that they are a higher presence.

Life—Yellow. It is spiritual in the beginning. It is bright white and resonates blue. It unites with yellow and creativity abounds. Your physicality is brought forth in bone and blood, mass and form. Life is at once matter and spirit.

Action—Green. Doing, being, producing, taking action is physical. It is the movement of thought, it is the direct order of vision. It is the footsteps of success. Action is a Choice and it brings about Change.

Solid—Blue. Solid is lessons learned. It is frozen time, frozen spirit. Solid is achievement. The medicines used to obtain solid are confidence and truth. Solid is truly a test of the Blue and Red Roads.

Full—Purple. Full is enough. Full is Complete. Full is an expansion and receiving of energy. It is the physical ability to know that spiritual is at hand, and you are complete within your project or your desire.

Worthy—Burgundy. Worthy is spiritual abundance brought forth in physical existence. It is the ability to look ahead and see, allowing that sight to direct you in your life as a pathway. Worthy is bestowed upon yourself from Knowledge, it is given to you by others out of Respect. Worthy is a necessity in order to achieve and appreciate Grand within the self.

HERBS

Cedar—Connects with Great Spirit, balances fear and anger by bringing about a cleansing of the spirit. Cedar oils stabilize, and cedar smoke blesses and enriches.

Cornmeal—Used to set sacred intention. It balances energy fields by anchoring and grounding. You can use cornmeal to feed spirit guides and spirit helpers. When you place it around the area where you are working, it welcomes spirits of light into your ceremony.

Juniper—Brings about protection when it is used as smoke or oil. It removes negative energy and creates an intense feeling. Be careful not to take too much juniper smoke into your lungs.

Piñon—Can be used in oil and as smoke. Piñon can be used as a protection herb to provide safety to your spirit and your physicality. It cleans and clears out negative energy, and invites the spirit world to listen and to speak.

Sage—An herb that freshens and cleanses the spirit. It demagnetizes negative energy and clears the aura. It cleans and brings about healing and honor within the self.

Sandalwood—Used for psychic ability. It opens, clears, and centers you. It allows you to see the spirit world very clearly, bringing about the ability to learn from your ancestors.

Sweet grass—A balancing herb that energizes, clears, and centers you. It is burned at sacred times and when you need strength. It reduces anxiety.

ANIMAL GUIDES AND TOTEMS

Ant—The keeper of full. One who knows, who is patient and who has all.

Bat—The keeper of obedience. The ability to laugh, to be able to see all situations, to fly quietly in your thoughts.

Bear—Teacher of introspection. Allows you to understand maturity and is the medicine of the relationship with self.

Cougar—A red medicine helper, guide, or totem. Cougar shows you the ability to Nurture, to protect, and to provide safety for your physical family as well as your spiritual being.

Crow—The keeper of the lesson of solid, the representation of listening to the ancestor within the spirit world.

Deer—Change. The deer is quiet and beauty. It is agile. It reminds us of our faith, the ability to look beyond and believe.

Dragon—The keeper of the lesson of purpose. A secret holder, one who stands back, who is mysterious. One who is hard to find. The energy of learning and bringing forth.

Fox—The symbol of Proof. It holds within its teeth the sharpness of truth. In its beauty it allows us to see that healing comes from swiftness. Its endurance and cleverness brings out our ability to perceive.

Human being—The master and keeper of the lesson of life. The being of opportunity, of senses, and feeling. The one who guards the doorway to the voice of the spirit through mental paths.

Ladybug—She is round: therefore she is the beginning and the end. You can divide her in half and divide that half in half—the ladybug walks as a medicine wheel. She speaks of the Ceremony of Life for she is the ambassador, she is the medicine who treats Life. She treats it with joy and patience. She treats it with the voice of the red star.

Lynx—The keeper of worthy. A quiet spirit, one who walks with knowledge, one who is Grand, with integrity. One who carries that in an open and honest way.

Ram—It is Grand, lofty, high-natured, noble, and proud. It is intense and accurate.

Raven—The one who protects and guides all spiritual activities. It is a voice of spirit, an ambassador of magic. It brings about your inner truth and gives you a natural ability to make a clear Choice.

Skunk—Speaks of black and white, an argument between fact and fiction. It does not fear, for it has no fierceness. It simply fights with its smell. It is wise to know that there is no need for violence. It holds within itself power with simply an aroma. It is the guide and symbol of peace. The black and white tells the story of Choice. The skunk gives the opportunity to strive without destruction and violence. It is Real within itself.

MINERAL MEDICINES

Agate—Used to awaken your talents. It brings about an understanding of self, strengthens the sight, and diminishes thirst. It helps you to communicate with the spiritual purpose of your physical cellular structure. It promotes inspiration and connects your physical mind and the spiritual world.

Amethyst—It is a stone of satisfaction, a stone of spirituality. It facilitates Change, brings about moderation, and works with the principles of metamorphosis, stability, invigoration, and perfect peace.

Aquamarine—A stone of courage. It stimulates and cleanses the voice, and the movements of speech. It promotes gentleness and moderation.

Beryl—Instills guidance in all sources of life. It enhances your physical individuality. It brings about independence, thought, and action.

Cat's Eye—Will give you great strengths and luck. It will enhance your awareness, and enable you to move out the unwanted energy of negative thoughts. It is protection energy that helps you focus on having clear spiritual sight.

Chrysocolloa—Helps to produce stability within the body. It can help you balance the blood sugar and strengthen your muscular structure. It stimulates your crown chakra. It can be used to purify your home and your environment. It promotes harmony, removes distress, and brings about great inner strength.

Citrine—A stabilizing stone used to balance your yin/yang energy. It also helps you to align the chakras and the ethereal planes.

Crystal—Known in many forms. It is quartz and is used for generating, promoting, enhancing, visioning, settling, calming, intensifying your emotions, solidifying your physicality, soothing, and calming.

Garnet—The stone of health. It is known to enhance Purpose; it enables the attitudes of devotion and helps to stabilize moods of abandonment. It allows one to connect with the inner self and brings freshness to the self.

Gold—Attracts the energy of physicality. It is a substance that is used to obtain material substance and prosperity.

Jasper (Picture)—This is a stone of universal, global, and world awareness. It promotes brother and sisterhood and helps us to work to save our planet.

Opal—Helps to invoke vision. It is a stone carried to enhance your ability to work with dreamtime. Often known as the stone of happy dreams and Changes, it can assist and allow you to become invisible in circumstances in which you do not want to be noticed.

Peridot—This stone is one that helps regulate cycles—physical, mental, and emotional. It provides a shield of protection for the body and can remove fear. It is a stone that helps the bruised ego. It helps you put yourself in order to move on to the next task.

Ruby, Raw—Promotes connectedness, protection, clearing, and strengthening of the mind.

Sapphire—A stone of prosperity. It brings about focus and regulates energy, broadening your horizons. It is often known as a form of star, the closest thing to a star's presence in physical form. It promotes beauty and expands your mind to understand your own beauty and intuition. It brings light-heartedness, joy, and a deepening of thought.

Silver—A substance that allows you to be in contact with Great Spirit, honoring and embracing Great Spirit, and protecting the totality of the self.

COLORS

Red—Confidence, strength, Nurture, color, accountability, patience, clarity, purpose, absolute, illumination, beginning.

Orange—Balance, success, Choice, energy, responsibility, unity, poise, obedience, correct, following, proceeding.

Yellow—Creativity, vision, Ceremony, prayer, sincerity, original, discipline, life, ideal, solid.

Green—Growth, beauty, Change, quiet, honesty, faith, account, action, flow, innocence.

Blue—Truth, healing, Proof, tranquility, respect, serenity, fact, solid, clear, introspection, understanding.

Purple—Wisdom, power, Real, knowledge, committed, reason, sense, full, depth.

Burgundy—Impeccability, great, Grand, will, mystery, worthy, worth, complete, spiritual, the path.

White—Silver, spiritual, All.

Black—Gold, totality, wholeness, physical, monetary, mass, material.

INDEX

Abandonment, 110, 186
Abuse, 148, 170
Acceptance, 86, 120
   teachings of, 49–50
Action, 14, 183
   elements, 96
   lesson of, 121–123
Actual, 123
Adaptability, 86
Agate, 185
Aging, 114
Alcoholic, 148
Altar, 133
Amethyst, 185
Analysis, 42
Animal guides and totems, 162, 184–185
Animation, 102
Ant, 13, 184
   teachings, 150–151
Antelope, 13
Aquamarine, 185
Aura, 103, 183
Balance, 186
Balancing herb, 184
Banishing herb, 31
Bat, 13, 68, 74, 184
   medicine, 85–87
Battle, 122
Beads, 163
Bear, 35–50, 184
   clan, 38
Beauty, 186
Being, 103
Beliefs, 49
Beryl, 185
Big Music, 22, 36–41, 156
Black, 187
   Horse, 126
   widow, 109
Blood, 49, 132, 156
Blue, 49, 187
   Road, 11, 13, 23, 41, 100, 138
   test of, 183
Blue–Eyed Raven, 72, 142
Bobcat, 112, 174
Body, 49
   balancing your, 132
Bodyworker, 120
Bone People, 19–25, 106, 108, 128, 156
Bones, 49, 132, 140
   talking, 124–138
Boundaries, 138
Bowl, water, 133–134

Brain, 49, 132; waves, 156
Breath, 49, 103
Burgundy, 49, 187
Burning incenses, 31
Cactus water, 134
Call of the Wolf, 168
Candles, 101
Careful, 77
Cat's Eye, 185
Cause, 65
Cedar, 183
Cells, 49
Ceremonial Medicine Pouch of the West, 83–85
Ceremonial Stick, 98–100
Ceremonial Water Bowl, 133–134
Ceremonialist, 98
Ceremony, 12, 27, 88–104, 134, 181, 186
   horse of, 177–178
Ceremony of the
   Breath of Life, 132–133
   Broken Stick of Forgiveness, 79–83
   Choice, 79–83
   Cleansing of the Physical Body, 116–121
   Connecting the Spirit and the Physical, 60–62
   Death, 110
   Five Colored Horses, 175–178
   Grandness, 161
   Intention, 45–47
   Introspection, 41–44
   Life, 84, 94
   Light, 100–102
   Sacred Herbs, 30–31
   Tree of Real, 148–150
   White Wolf, 178–179
   Worthy, 164–167
Chakras, 49, 103
Chance, 108, 112
Change, 12, 17, 77, 108, 109, 111, 112, 121–123, 182, 183, 184, 187
   stone of, 186
   teachings of, 113–116
Choice, 12, 27, 57–58, 67–69, 73, 76, 79–80, 95, 109, 181, 182, 183, 185, 187
   teachings of, 77–78
Chrysocolloa, 185
Citrine, 185
Clan color, 99

Cleansing the spirit, stone for, 183
Cleansing the physical body, 116–121
Color, 97
Colors, 49, 158
   spiritual, 48–49
Complete, 12, 137, 144
Confidence, 186
Cornmeal, 183
Cougar, 13, 52, 184
   medicine, 59–60
Council of Grand, 153, 155
Counsel, 42
Counseling, 120, 161
Courage, stone of, 185
Coyote, King, 91
Creativity, 182, 186
Crow, 13, 184
   teachings, 134–138
Crown chakra, stone to stimulate, 185
Crystal, 186
Dark Eyes, 52, 76, 94, 110–112, 125, 128–129, 141–143, 153–155, 175
Death, 38–41, 52, 125–126, 138, 141
   spirit of, 52
Decision, make a, 47
Deer, 13, 184
   Fading Deer, 109, 154
   White–Tailed, 113
   Woman, 109, 111–112, 143
Deliberation, 42
Depression, 148
Devotion, 64, 65
Different, 114
Direction, 46
Directions, 133
Discernment, 78, 181
Dismissal, 79–83
DNA, 27, 49, 132
Dragon, 13, 57, 184
Dreams, stone of happy, 186
Dreamtime, 175, 186
   horse of, 177
Drug abuse, 148
E.G., 68, 73–76, 105, 112
Effect, 123
Elders, 135–136, 154
Elements, the, 97
Elk Man, 154
Emotions, 13, 150
   section of wheel, 11
End in view, 46

189

Energetic, 122
Energy, 13, 49, 132
   fields, 49, 103
   the story holder, 156
Evil, 74, 85–87, 148
Examination, 42, 45
Excellent, 137
Existence, 102–103
Fading Deer, 109, 154
Faithfulness, 87
Fear, 85–86, 109, 110
   to remove, 186
Feelings, 13, 103
Fine, 137
Fire Heart, 156
Flesh, 49
Flow, 34
Fluids in body, 49
Footprints, 148
Force, 103
Forgiveness, 79–83
Form, 49
Fourteen, 138
Fox, 13, 184
   Dancer, 131
   Medicine, 130–131
Foxes, 128
Frame, 49
Friends, 74–75
Full, 183
   lesson of, 150–151
Garnet, 186
Gentleness, 87
Give, 114
Give–away, 45, 62, 80, 101, 115
Goals, 62, 138; setting, 45–46
God, Voice of, 22
Gold, 186
Golden Door, 143, 152–167
Golden Heart, 53, 54, 58
Grand, 12, 27, 160, 182, 187
   Council, 153, 158
Grandfather Wolf, see Wolf
Grandmother Moon, 146
Grand Ram, 158
Gratitude, 133, 151
Great Spirit, 140, 167
   herb to contact, 183
   stone of contact with, 186
Green, 49, 121, 187
Grief, 52, 53, 57
Grim Reaper, 126
Growth, 186
Guidance, stone to provide, 185
Habits, bad, 119–120, 178–179
Hair, 49
Handprints, 149

Healer, 117
Healing
   color that promotes, 187
   stone that brings about, 183
Health
   good, 122
   searching, 42
   stone of, 186
Heartbeat, 103
Helen, 57
Herbs
   banishing, 31
   healing, 31
   see Ceremony of the Sacred Hoop, sacred, 14
Horse, black, 126
Horses, colored, 170
   see Ceremony of the Five
Human, 13, 184
   teachings of the, 102–104
Immortality, 182
Impeccability, 87, 187
Incenses, burning, 31
Intention
   Ceremony of, 45–47
   questions of, 47
   spiritual, 183
Introspection, 38, 40, 41
   Ceremony of, 41–44
   teacher of, 184
Invisibility, 186
Jasper (picture), 186
Journal, 25–26
Journey, 12
Judge, 138
Juniper, 183
Keeper of Obedience, 184
Keeper of Full, 184
Keeper of Purpose, 57
Keeper of Solid, 184
Keeper of the lesson of life, 184
Keeper of Worthy, 184
Keepers of the West
   see Raven
   see Big Music
King Coyote, 91, 168
Knowledge, 86, 151
Ladybug, 13, 89–91, 93, 184; medicine, 96–98
Lesson words, 182–183
Lessons, the Seven Sacred, 12
Letting go, 79
Life, 12, 49, 114, 182
   Circles, 60–62
   lesson of, 102–104
Love, 141
Luck, stone of, 185

Lynx, 13, 184
   teachings, 164
Magic, 98
Marriage, 97, 136, 137
Medicine, 133
   blanket, 28
   Pouch, Ceremonial, 83–85
   wheel, 11, 92, 114
   words, 181–182
Medicines
   the Seven Sacred, 12, 27
   Memory, 156
Mind, 49, 156, 175
   sections of wheel, 11
Mineral medicines, 185–186
Miracle, 98
Moon medicine, 24
Moving, 122–123
Mule Deer, teachings of the, 121–123
Muscular structures, 49, 132
Mystery, 86
Nails, 49
Nerves, 49
Neuro–processes within the brain, 49, 132
North Wind, 38
Nurture, 181, 186
Nurture, 12, 27, 52–53, 181, 186
   bundle, 62–64
   spirit keeper of, 53
   teachings of, 59–60
Obedience, 12, 68–69, 73, 105, 182, 186
   lesson of, 85–87
Old Bone Man and Woman, 19–25
Old Woman Rock, 14, 55–58, 68, 91–94, 153
Opal, 186
Opportunity, 12, 78, 86, 91, 123, 126
   horse of, 176
Orange, 49, 182, 186
   balance, 150
   medicine, 150
   Stars, 75
Organs, 49
Ownership, 112
Parenting, 115
Passivity, 87
Perform, 122
Physical
   Bone, Horse of, 176
   existence, 48–49
   lessons of, 12
   medicine bundle, 62–64
   sections of wheel, 11
   wholeness, 119

Physicality, keeper of/see Big Music
Piñon, 183
Pole, ceremonial, 98–100
Politeness, 97–98
Pouches, 162
Power, 78
Prayer, 93, 101
  ties, 28–30
Principle, 65
Process of the Lesson of Worthy, 164
Project organization, 46
Proof, 12, 73, 182
  circle of, 128–130
  teachings of, 130–131
Prosperity, stone of, 186
Protection, 183, 186
  Horse of, 177
Protein, 49
Psychic ability, stone to enhance, 184
Pumpkin, 172
Purple, 49, 187
Purpose, 12, 45, 57, 59, 72, 182, 186
  lesson of, 64–66
Quartz, 186
Rainbow Medicine, 11–12
  teachings of the West, 26
  totem and guide teachings, 183–187
  Wheel, 11, 31–34
Ram, 13, 185
  Grand, 158
Raven, 13, 74, 76, 85–86, 111, 112, 184
  Blue–Eyed, 72, 170
  medicine, 77–78
Real, 12, 27, 143, 182, 187
  and reality, 139–140
  teachings of, 139–151
  tree of, 144
Reason, 66
Red, 49, 186
  medicine, 59, 64
  Red Road, 11, 13, 23, 41, 100, 136
  test of, 183
Reflection, 43
Remodel, 115
Reproduction, 103
Resilience, 103
Respect, 87, 97
Ribbons, 132
Right, 77
Roads, Red and Blue, 11
Rock, 91; Old Woman, see Old Woman Rock

Sacred, 98
  Hoop of Life, 126
Sadness, 109
Sage, 183
Sandalwood, 184
Seasons of life, 131
Selection, 78
Self–confidence, 41
Self–esteem, 41
Shamanism, 12, 13, 14
Shaman's necklace, 162–163
Shenonna Woman, 144
Sicknesses, 117–118, 133
Silver, 186
Silverware, 144
Sister, 89, 93
  see Wildflower
Skeleton, 19, 49
  spirit, 159
Skins, 49
Skunk, 13, 185
  medicine, 144–148
  Woman, 144
Smudging, 30–31
  see Ceremony of the Sacred Herbs
Snake Man, 58, 68, 75, 95, 105–109, 125
Soft Spirit, 36
Solemn, 97
Solid, 12, 183
  lesson of, 134–138
Song, the, 111
Song of Great Spirit, 12
Song of the Bones, 139–151
Soul, 49
  searching, 43
Sphere, 85
Spider, 109
  sacred, 143
Spiral, life as, 103
Spirit, 13, 49, 65, 103, 132, 156
  lessons of, 11
  school of, 23
  section of wheel, 11
Spirit, Great, 140
Spirits, light, 155–159
Spiritual
  colors, 48
  connection with, 119
Spirituality, stone of, 185
Stabilizing stone, 185
Standing Bear, 38
Star people, 106
Stars as colors, 48
Steadfastness, 66

Stick
  broken, 79–83
  ceremonial, 98–100
  Woman, 169–175
Strength, 181
  stones to provide, 184, 185
Strict, 97
Sturdy, 137
Success, 186
Sun, moon and seven stars, 11, 17
Survival, 110
Sweet grass, 184
Talents, stone to awaken, 185
Talking
  Bones, 124–138
  Circle, 153
Temperature, 49
Thought, 13, 49, 103
Tissues, 49
Totems, 13
Touch, 106
Transform, 115–116
Tree of Real, 148–150
Truth, 23, 85, 110, 187
Truths, pointing out, 147
Understanding yourself, 41–44
Undertaking, 122
Uniqueness, 123, 124
Veins, 49
Vision, 11, 46, 65, 181, 186
Vital principle, 49
Voice of Creator, 22, 36
Water, 49
  bowl, 133–134
West, keeper of the
  see Big Music
White, 187
White–Tailed Deer, 113
Wholeness, 150
Wildflower, 92–93
Wind, Voice of the, 88–104
Wolf, 74, 85–86
Wolf, Grandfather, 112–113
  Grandmother and Grandfather, 17–20, 21, 24, 94–96
  medicine, 152
  White, 75–76, 178–179
  Woman medicine, 24
Words, 13
Worth, 160
Worthy, 12, 78, 183
  lesson of, 164
Yellow, 49, 186
Yin/yang balance, 185

191

To find out about conferences and workshops,
or to contact the author, visit our website:
www.wolfmoondanceauthor.com
Or write:

Wolf Moondance
453 East Wonderview Avenue
P.O. Box 6000
Estes Park, CO 80517